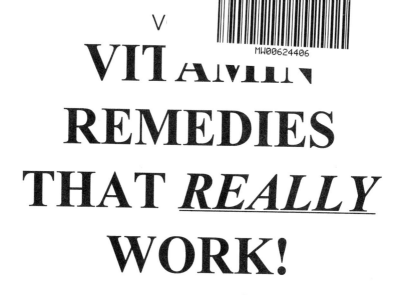

VITAMIN REMEDIES THAT _REALLY_ WORK!

Safe Easy Directions For Healing And Preventing
Over 50 Common Conditions

LYNN CAPEHART, J.D.

CRICKET PUBLISHING GROUP
P.O. Box 90458
San Diego, California, 92169

All rights reserved under International and Pan-American Copyright Conventions. Published in the United States by Cricket Publishing Group

Library of Congress Card Catalog Number: 99-93302

ISBN 0-9672552-0-1

Manufactured in the United States of America
First Cricket Publishing Group Trade Edition: January 2000

Cover Photo: Brian Goodloe
Author's Makeup: Michellemarie Hutton, Lorac Cosmetics

ATTENTION Colleges, Universities, Medical Schools, Teaching Hospitals, HMOs, Insurance Companies, Corporations, and Professional Organizations: Quantity discounts are available on bulk purchases of this book for educational or training purposes, non-profit fund raising, or gift giving. For information please contact: Marketing Department, Cricket Publishing Group, P.O.B. 90458, San Diego, California, 92169.

This volume is dedicated to

Mary Grace, the grandmother who taught me to respect myself,

Raleigh, the father who taught me courage,

Lucille, the mother I lost who taught me trust,

Maryann, the aunt who taught me fairness to others, and

Charlie, mentor, who showed me how high soars the generous spirit.

ACKNOWLEDGMENTS

I want to thank my faithful editors for their committed participation and unflagging enthusiasm, even in the face of early morning phone calls, when I couldn't wait to get an answer to yet another burning question.

Uwanna Thomas, M.B.A., Cmdr. U.S. Navy Res.
Marie Backes, J.D.
Mary DeYoung, J.D.
Jaqui Parker, R.Ph.
Greg Paniccia, M.D.
Susan Backes

A heartfelt thank you to all my subjects, who trusted me enough to try the remedies and cared enough to report back with the results.

I also owe a debt of gratitude to all my readers, who commented on individual chapters of the manuscript, and to those who made other valuable contributions to the book.

Millie Backes
Anna Blecksmith
Edie Boulet
J. D. Crow
Ann Smitz Davis
Ernest Echaves
Robert I. Fox, M.D.
Mary Garrison
Al Hardac
Julie A. Heck
Rhomie L. Heck, III
Rosalynne Whitaker-Heck, M.S.
Thea Heinz
Beth Henney, R.Ph., J.D.
Larry Hermansen
Al Irvine
Laila W. Keith
Tish Kraft, J.D.

Richard W. Lindsay, D.M.D.
Ann Munsey
The New Seed, San Diego
Linda Nickell, Ph.D.
Nordstrom Fashion Valley,
  San Diego
Samuel D. Osowski, M.B.A., J.D.
Yvonne Pasternak
People's Food Coop, San Diego
Sherree Ramirez
David Rubincam
Charles Shockley, Ph.D.
Barbara Silkworth, M.A.
Sharon Pettey Taylor, M.S., M.A.
Angelique Torres
Vivian M. Warfield, M.A.
Yvonne Ladson Webb

Here Is What People Are Saying About The Remedies In VITAMIN REMEDIES THAT *REALLY* WORK!

"I work twelve-hour night shifts caring for sick babies. It is a joyous and rewarding career but very tiring. No matter how much I used to sleep, I could never shake that groggy feeling. This is a common complaint among my coworkers. It got so bad that on days off I basically didn't want to get out of bed and function normally. After a week on Lynn's CoQ10 and Vitamin B12 remedy, I began to feel better. As time passed, my stamina increased. Now I have two jobs, and I work out four times a week. I feel healthier now though I'm working twice as hard."

Rita Lahr, R.N.
Neonatal Intensive Care
UCSD Medical Center
San Diego

"I used this remedy for preventing hangovers when I was in college. Before going to a party, my classmates and I would load up on the L-Cysteine and C Complex combo. Instead of nursing a hangover the next day, we all felt fine and were able to study and work. In fact, if I took enough of the combo I didn't even get intoxicated."

Lisa Kraig
Administrative Assistant
Queens, N.Y.

"My job began really tiring me out by the end of the day. On top of a grueling law enforcement schedule, I elected to take on the additional learning curve of flight training. At Lynn's recommendation, I started a regimen of Coenzyme Q10, Gingko Biloba and L-Glutamine. Within two weeks, I noticed that my stamina and ability to retain and quickly recall information had improved quite impressively. I got my pilot's license in record time!"

David M. Rubincam
Special Agent FBI, Seattle

"As the primary care giver for a mother with Alzheimer's, I

found the remedies in this book astonishing. After just three weeks on the remedy, I noticed a difference in her temperament. After ten months I had my mother back. The improvement in her condition has taken away much of the stress I bore in caring for her. This book contains miracles."

Mrs. Gloria Thomas
Retail Sales, Newport News, Va.

"I have lived with debilitating asthma since the day I was born. I gave up my inhaler after just six weeks on this book's treatment."

Taylor Bowman
English Teacher
New York City

"I hurt my hand water skiing and had to have a joint replaced. My doctor said it would take two months for the wound to heal completely. I didn't begin the Beta Carotene remedy until after surgery. When I returned for a post-op appointment, the wound had healed so well--with no sign of a scar--that I played a game and challenged my doctor to find the finger joint on which he operated. He couldn't! He actually had to check my chart because there was nothing about my hand to indicate I'd had major surgery three weeks earlier. Beta Carotene is truly miraculous."

Susan Backes
Sales Consultant, San Diego

"I have suffered from migraine and tension headaches for most of my life, sometimes three to four times a week. Even though I am a physician I could not find a prescription drug that prevented them. But my headaches stopped after only three weeks taking the daily remedy found in Lynn's book. As long as I take it I have no problems."

Greg Paniccia, M.D., Director of Research
Charter/API Hospital Psychiatric Health Systems
San Diego

"My husband John had two operations on the same hip. For the first operation we didn't use Beta Carotene; three years later the scar is still rough to touch, welted, humped, and just horrible looking. For the second operation John took Beta Carotene daily. His recovery for the second operation was remarkable: Even though the second incision was larger than the first, it took much less time to heal, and the wound was not as sensitive. We are amazed at the difference in the two scars. The second one is a smooth thin line without welting that continues to fade.

Mary Garrison
Hospital Volunteer and Homemaker
Rancho Penasquitos, Ca.

"I have smoked cigarettes for over 30 years, sometimes a half pack a day. I often felt congestive and had a "cottony" feeling in my lungs at the end of the day. Since I have been following this vitamin remedy I breathe much easier, and my lungs are clearer."

Vivian M. Warfield, M.A.
Arts Administrator/Musician
New York City

"As a pharmacist I am on my feet ten to twelve hours a day, several days a week. I often experienced spontaneous bruising on my legs. I was worried that this condition might indicate week blood vessel walls, and that it could lead to varicose veins. I began following the Rutin remedy and was amazed at the results. It really works. Since I have been taking it everyday, I no longer suffer leg bruising."

Jaqui Parker, R.Ph.
Pharmacist, Barrington, R.I.

"I injured a knee tendon while playing football with my three sons. My doctor said the injury would take several months to heal properly and prescribed daily aspirin. I hobbled around on a cane for two weeks feeling a lot of pain. I even had to sit down to play my bass during performances. Then I tried the Beta Carotene remedy. Six days later I tossed the cane because my leg was totally healed. I wish I hadn't waited."

Simon "Bigga" Echaves
Musician/Composer
National City, Ca.

GREGORY PANICCIA, M.D.

Health care in the United States has been in a state of flux for over a decade. During that time, many patients and health care professionals have often felt they were relinquishing control of the important decisions regarding the doctor-patient relationship and individual treatment. In this atmosphere, it is easy for the average person to get the feeling that they are no longer in control of their own health.

One great thing about Vitamin Remedies That _Really_ Work! is that it gives you not only the sense, but the reality, of having more control over your own health. Dr. Capehart gives you that control in easy to follow remedies for some of the most common ailments of our time. She writes in the simplest of terms and manages to convey a great deal of information in a short space, something every reader will appreciate. Her remedies are nonintrusive, inexpensive, and can offer many people a safe effective alternative to drug treatments that don't work, or that have unpleasant side effects. I know this personally, because I had suffered from migraine and tension headaches for years--and couldn't find a drug that worked--until I followed Dr. Capehart's recommendations. And you know what? I no longer get them.

Another bonus is the short story at the end of each chapter that makes the remedy so much easier to remember. The stories actually divert you and are good enough to stand on their own outside the book. You wouldn't expect a book of this kind to be so entertaining. Health books are not supposed to entertain you, only educate, but Vitamin Remedies That _Really_ Work! does both, remarkably well.

i

JAQUI PARKER, R.Ph.

We have all experienced events in life that hit us right between the eyes. Forevermore, your life, or your perception of life, is changed. And then there are those events which can only be seen, and fully appreciated, with hindsight. Life changed, you just didn't know it at the time. Encountering the information Dr. Capehart shares in this book falls into the latter category.

As both a health care professional and a consumer, I have found Vitamin Remedies That *Really* Work! to be an invaluable resource. I didn't know when she started sharing her knowledge with me that I would personally employ it as extensively as I have. What surprises me even more is how often I have drawn from this resource to give my pharmacy patients an alternative remedy for some of the most common ailments. I would never dream of sharing these remedies with patients if I didn't completely trust their validity and safety.

The important information accumulated in this book is only one part of its great value. After a very clear, easy-to-follow description of each remedy, Dr. Capehart creates a wonderfully alive story which illustrates the use of that remedy. A good analogy would be to consider the health information as a nutritional dinner followed by a fine, flavorful dessert--the vignette. These stories capture your attention so completely that you are compelled to read to the end. What a surprise! a health book that you simply cannot put down! An unexpected, but much appreciated, by-product of this unique format is that the story will help you remember the remedy. You meet a character, are intrigued in some way, and easily remember the related remedy.

For anyone interested in safe effective remedies for common ailments--*this is a book to own.* For anyone simply interested in good storytelling--*this is a book to own.*

PREFACE

Why This Book Is Different From Any Vitamin Book Ever Written

---

Vitamin Remedies That _Really_ Work! is the only book that tells you *how to use* natural food supplements to heal and prevent common medical conditions. It is the only book that tells you precisely what supplement to take, for which ailment, how much to take, and how often to take it. It is the only book that tells you exactly what results to expect and gives you a time frame in which to expect them. Perhaps best of all, it assumes that the reader knows nothing about how to use supplements as remedies, so the directions are simple, step-by-step, hold-my-hand instructions that are impossible to misunderstand.

Many vitamin books give you more information than you want, but still do not tell you exactly *how to use* a supplement to treat a specific condition. That is all this book will tell you. If you are looking for more information on supplements, you will have to look elsewhere. This book does not contain information you do not need in order to use a supplement as a remedy. You will find no complex historical data here. No technical information on recommended daily allowances. No confusing details about what foods contain which supplements. And there are no diets or recipes. Instead, this is a simple, hands-on, "how to" book, with easy access to brief instructions telling you what you need to know to use supplements to treat illness: And everything you need to know to use a supplement as a remedy is found in this book.

The alphabetical **Cross Reference** and **Index** give you quick access to the remedies for all the conditions addressed, as well as, an overview of supplements used. The **Remedy At A Glance Charts** in each chapter make it easy to reference a remedy without rereading the instructions each time.

Each chapter concludes with a case study written as an entertaining and inspirational short story about someone who uses the remedy to heal and prevent a medical condition. You can relate to these people no matter who you are because they share the same problems as

v

you. They are women and men, old and young, black and white, rich and poor, single and married. The stories take place in various locations like New York, San Diego, Dallas, the Midwest, Seattle, Los Angeles, Aspen, Puerto Rico, France, and Mexico.

These personal accounts relate to the human condition and do more than just entertain. They make it easier to remember the directions in the first part of the chapter. You may forget Ginkgo Biloba and L-Glutamine, but you will remember Moshe, the kosher deli owner in Manhattan who uses the combination to recover his super memory. Or Betsy, the ninety-two year old granddaughter of a slave, who uses Vitamin B12 to help her outpace her forty-something nephew during a visit to San Diego's Sea World. To protect their privacy, pseudonyms have been used for most of the subjects of the case studies, and non-relevant biographical details have been changed. Real names are used in the personal testimonials found on the front pages. All of these people used supplements to help them reach their "Maximum Best". You can use their experiences to help you reach your own.

The "Maximum Best" Philosophy

The intellectual foundation of **Vitamin Remedies That _Really_ Work!** is the **"Maximum Best Philosophy"**, which embodies the principle of living responsibly and includes a duty to the _self_--to try to fully realize your own potential. Maximum Best is completely personal. You can no more compare your Maximum Best to another person's than you can compare your fingerprints. It involves letting go of the world, the outside competition, and looking inside to compete with yourself. In other words, you can only gauge your attainment of Maximum Best by competing with yourself.

One problem with competing with other people as a way of measuring your own abilities is that you are constantly dependent on--and limited to--the quality of the competition. If you win a race against people whose abilities are far below yours, it can be an empty victory. And there is no disgrace in placing last when you are outclassed by the competition--if you reached _your_ Maximum Best in trying. If you could fast forward to the end of your life and look back, your Maximum Best would be the highest points you reached in your lifetime. Maximum Best is better than your best. It is a level you must reach and stretch and tax to attain. Some people reach it a couple of times a week, others only once in a lifetime. Everyone has a Maximum Best even if he or she reaches it rarely.

Illness is one variable that will affect your ability to attain Maximum Best; healing and preventing illness with food supplements is the focus of this book. Your body's warning plus your timely response *can* equal prevention, making it possible to age without severe illness, but if you do not take care of your health, your body and mind will retaliate against you as you age. Consider the serious debilitations-- preventable cancers, ruined livers, broken-down kidneys, worn-out hearts, fused and arthritic joints, deformed spines, clogged arteries and confused minds--which could be avoided by making responsible choices about your health now.

Naturally, you cannot account for or control every genetic predisposition to a specific condition, but you can do more to heal yourself than you have been led to believe. With the unique information contained in **Vitamin Remedies That _Really_ Work!**, you have the power, right now, to heal and prevent many potentially debilitating conditions. For most people, the natural treatments can produce astonishing results in a short period of time and are fairly inexpensive when compared with drug treatments. If you follow the instructions carefully, the supplements can improve, suppress, heal, and even prevent the conditions they address.

*   *   *

Please write to me if you discover any new uses for these or other supplements. Also, I would be interested in knowing the results you achieve when using the remedies as directed. If you agree, your information may be passed along in Volume II so that others may benefit. Good health and good reading.

Dr. Lynn Capehart
San Diego, California

TABLE OF CONTENTS

CHAPTER 1

21 THINGS YOU NEED TO KNOW BEFORE YOU USE THE REMEDIES IN THIS BOOK

---

1. The remedies in this book are based on a belief that the human body is a single universe where the same physical laws pertain, no matter where in that universe they are applied. That is why a clog or blockage anywhere in the body will respond to essentially the same treatment, whether in an artery, a joint, a heart valve, a lung, or gout in a big toe. Likewise, infection or inflammation anywhere will respond to the same treatments, because the body is a single, interactive system that can be stimulated by the remedies to utilize the appropriate mechanism to repair itself, regardless of where an injury or illness is located.

2. Read *all* directions before using a supplement as a remedy. Each supplement or combination of supplements is covered in one chapter. The first part of the chapter contains the directions and all information you need to use the supplement as a remedy. The second part is a case study written as a short story about someone who uses the remedy to overcome a medical problem. These personal accounts are entertaining and will help you understand how the supplement works, but it is not necessary that you read them. You should read and follow all the instructions in the first part if you want to be successful using the supplement as a remedy.

3. Make sure you understand all the instructions before taking a supplement. Ask yourself: In what form should you buy the supplement--tablets, capsules, softgels? Which strength formula should you buy? How many times a day and in what dosage is it taken? When is it taken--morning, afternoon or evening? Is there a maximum daily dosage you should not exceed? Does the daily dosage vary from day to day or week to week? Do you need a "therapeutic dose" or only a "maintenance dose"? Can the supplement be taken with liquids only or is food necessary? Does it have to be taken simultaneously with any other supplements to be effective? What is the time frame for achieving results? Which brands did the author use? These are the questions you need answered before using a remedy. All of the answers are contained in the following chapters.

4. If you have trouble swallowing a supplement, try this method: Instead of using the liquid to *push* the supplement down your throat, place it in the middle of your tongue, let your mouth fill with liquid, and then swallow. The supplement should wash down your throat floating in the liquid without any problem.

5. You do not have to stop taking any medications in order to experience the benefits and healing effects of the supplement remedies. As you use a remedy over time, you will often find that you need less and less medication as the natural remedy heals your condition.

6. Although the chapter title lists the primary supplement(s) necessary to heal an ailment, in some instances the Notes√√ suggest additional supplements that can increase the benefits of a particular remedy. The additional supplements play an important role in assisting a primary remedy to heal a condition.

7. Sustained release or time-released formulas are not recommended, because the remedies will not be effective unless you can obtain the benefits of a full potency dose.

8. Often, the recommended daily doses exceed those of the U.S. Department of Agriculture, because it often takes large daily amounts of a supplement to effect a remedy. The supplements cannot and will not work therapeutically unless they are maintained in your system at sufficient levels and for sustained periods of time. The therapeutic doses produce the high blood levels and tissue saturation necessary for natural healing, and can be taken safely for days, weeks, or years at a time--depending on the severity of the condition. As long as your body is ailing and in need of the remedy it can accept the larger doses.

However, once your condition has healed be sure to follow the directions to stop or reduce to a "maintenance dose" to avoid creating an imbalance in your system. While proper dosage is crucial to the success of the natural treatments, it can be a mistake to exceed the suggested levels. If you do, the supplements will not be absorbed by your system; you will excrete them, or they may leech out other nutrients resulting in a different deficiency than the one being treated. You may even experience an allergic reaction.

9. It takes smaller daily amounts of a supplement to prevent a recurrence of a condition once it has been brought under control. This "maintenance dose" is taken daily to prevent the initial onset of a condition--and to prevent a prior-healed condition from returning. If you are treating a temporary illness, the directions give you the option of stopping the supplement.

10. If your symptoms return or worsen after reducing your dosage, at any time during the healing process, either repeat the entire procedure starting at step one, or simply return to the next highest dosage that brought relief. In some cases the directions tell you to repeat the procedure by starting with step two instead of step one.

11. Generally, you must continue taking a supplement every day or the healing benefits you have gained will end shortly after you stop--much the same way you would lose the benefits of food if you were to stop eating. This is especially true for water soluble supplements that usually cannot be stored in the body. This means you may have to take supplements for the rest of your life to avoid certain conditions.

12. Your body's warning plus your timely response *can* equal prevention. If you learn to recognize the early warning signs of an illness, you can usually avoid the condition entirely. That means paying close attention to your body's signals and taking offensive measures in order to prevent the onset of an ailment. It is generally easier to avoid a condition than it is to heal it once it has invaded your body.

13. There are few side effects associated with using the remedies. Those that have been reported, such as nagging headaches or rashes, are minor, usually occur only in the first few weeks after beginning the remedy, and end immediately if the remedy is stopped. Usually, just lowering the dosage or interrupting treatment for a day will alleviate the problem.

14. You can experience other beneficial responses when using a remedy, besides healing the condition you are targeting. For instance, Lecithin used to clean out arthritic joints can also lower cholesterol, clean excess congestion from lungs, unclog arteries and heart valves without surgery, help dissolve gallstones, and end gout.

15. The supplements discussed in this book are not food replacements. They cannot fulfill the need for a balanced diet. You need the bulk, fiber, enzymes, and trace elements found in whole foods to be completely healthy *and* to properly absorb and utilize food supplements. Nutritionists continue to discover new supplements in whole foods of which we were previously unaware.

16. The supplements are easier to digest and absorb when taken with food. Though many are known to be "water soluble," it is not recommended that you take them with water alone. If you are taking supplements without food, try to use juice or other liquids that are more substantial than water. If the instructions are to take a supplement with food, it is important to do so whenever possible.

17. Drink at least eight ounces of liquids when taking supplements. Don't sip enough just to get them down. This is especially important if you are taking several supplements together. If you don't drink enough liquid, expect some stomach distress, heartburn, or other signs of indigestion. Any discomfort should ease immediately if you drink a glass of juice or other liquids. If not, eat a small portion of a complex carbohydrate--like a slice of bread. If you still have trouble digesting a particular supplement, try taking it with 400 mg of **Betaine Hydrochloride,** one of the digestive acids found in the stomach which is available as a supplement. You can also use vinegar mixed with water in an eight to one ratio (eight ounces of water to one ounce of vinegar), to alleviate the *worst* indigestion. Parents can use a twelve to one ratio for infants and toddlers.[1]

18. The nutritional supplements include vitamins, minerals, amino acids, herbs, and other organic formulations. They are used in the form of tablets, capsules, and softgels. *Tablets* are compressed solid. *Capsules* contain loose powder encased in a stiff gelatin mold and sometimes dissolve faster in the stomach than tablets. *Softgels* contain oil based supplements such as Beta Carotene in a soft gelatin mold. Due to a supplement's chemical components or intended use, one form may be recommended over another; be sure to use the recommended form. A choice is given where no perceived differences exist among the forms.

19. Many supplements act as natural diuretics and may increase urination. This is not cause for alarm because you will lose only excess water which may translate into the loss of a few pounds. Also, urine may be a deeper yellow after taking some daily remedies. This is due to the concentration of nutrients and is nothing to worry about.

20. The author has no financial connection or other

---

1 If your infant is dry, fed, and well, and still cries in distress for no apparent reason, consider that he or she may have indigestion. Most infant diets are largely starch and protein, very difficult substances to digest even for an adult stomach. They contain little or no fresh fruits and vegetables, and therefore not enough of the enzymes that are necessary for good digestion.

affiliation with the companies whose brands she uses. A brand is listed based on the author's experience in utilizing that particular one to achieve the desired results. In selecting a brand, careful consideration is given to the source of the ingredients, the formula strength, and whether the price is competitive.

21. Milligram (mg), and microgram (mcg) are both used in the text: 1 milligram equals 1000 micrograms.

CHAPTER 2

GINKGO BILOBA AND L-GLUTAMINE
Taken Together In Combination

•Treat Alzheimer's And Geriatric Dementia
Slowing And Reversing Their Ravaging Effects On Mental Capabilities

•Reverse Memory Loss
Regaining And Surpassing Your Prior Memory Capacity

•Improve Learning Abilities And Fight Mental Fatigue
Increasing Analytical Skills And Ability To Assimilate New Information

Ginkgo Biloba is an herb. L-Glutamine is an amino acid, one of the "building blocks" of protein. Taken together they can have a remarkable effect on mental capabilities and stamina, improving the brain's ability to learn, think, reason, and remember.

If you, or someone you care about, have been diagnosed with Alzheimer's or other form of geriatric dementia, Ginkgo Biloba and L-Glutamine can bring marked improvement within three to four weeks, regardless of how bad the condition is or how long the person has suffered from the problem. Improvement can be found in two areas: *cognitive*--in memory, judgment, and the ability to concentrate, as well as *behavioral*--in calmer temperament, less withdrawal, and greater ability to cope with the daily trials of living.

If normal forgetfulness is your problem, or if you are trying to learn difficult new information, the combination can enhance your mental abilities and cause them to increase over time, until they level off at your Maximum Best. If there has been actual memory loss, or if you are burned out and suffering from mental exhaustion, the combination can restore--and help you to exceed--your prior mental abilities. The increased mental proficiency can be sustained as long as you continue the remedy daily.

Recommended Strength[2]

Ginkgo Biloba--60 mg (Formula: 24%, 50:1 Standardized Extract)

L-Glutamine--500 mg

Recommended Form

Ginkgo Biloba--capsules only

L-Glutamine--tablets or capsules

Taken How

A Single Dose: 1 Ginkgo Biloba and 2 L-Glutamine (60 mg Ginkgo Biloba, and 1000 mg L-Glutamine) taken together, with eight ounces of juice or other liquids as directed.

---

2 The author has had the best results with NOW® Ginkgo Biloba, Glendale Hts, IL 60139, (800) 999-8069. For L-Glutamine, the best results have been obtained with Country Life®, Hauppauge, NY 11788, (800) 645-5768; Puritan's Pride®, Oakdale, NY 11769, (800) 645-1030; Solgar®, Leonia, NJ 07605, (800) 645-2246; and Twinlab®, Ronkonkoma NY 11779, (800) 645-5626. Puritan's Pride is available by mail order only. The other brands can be purchased at most health foods stores and sometimes in the health foods section of supermarkets.

Side Effects

Some brands of Ginkgo Biloba can cause headaches in some individuals. None reported with L-Glutamine when taken as directed.

Notes√√

√ Taken alone, these supplements will not have the desired therapeutic effect. They should be taken together--at the same time--to be effective as a remedy.

•Treat Alzheimer's And Geriatric Dementia

Slowing And Reversing Their Ravaging Effects On Mental Capabilities

1. Take a single dose of Ginkgo Biloba and L-Glutamine every four hours, i.e., 8:00 a.m., Noon, 4:00 p.m., and 8:00 p.m., and continue until your symptoms are gone.

2. Reduce to a single dose three times daily, morning, afternoon, and evening, and continue as a maintenance dose to help prevent the condition.

Remedy At A Glance (Ginkgo Bilboa And L-Glutamine)

	8:00 am	Noon	4:00 pm	8:00 pm
Daily To Relieve Symptoms:	Single Dose	Single Dose	Single Dose	Single Dose

	Morning	Afternoon	Evening
Daily As A Maintenance Dose:	Single Dose	Single Dose	Single Dose

Notes√√

√ Some improvement in temperament can be seen after just a few weeks. Other cognitive functions can show measurable improvement in as little as a month. These improvements can be maintained only as long as the recommended dosage is taken every day. Missing even one dose on a regular basis can cause an improved condition to deteriorate measurably.

√ Numerous recent studies have confirmed that **Vitamin E Complex** helps slow the mental deterioration associated with Alzheimer's and other forms of geriatric dementia. It is recommended that you add it to the Ginkgo Biloba and L-Glutamine.

Vitamin E Complex: Use in 400 IU softgels only, *mixed* tocopherols only.[3] Take it once a day with food as directed, regardless of the amount you are taking.

1. Take 1200 IU daily, and continue for four weeks.

2. Reduce to 800 IU daily, and continue as a maintenance dose to help support good mental health.

Remedy At A Glance (Vitamin E Complex)

	Once A Day
Daily For One Month To Relieve Symptoms:	1200 IU
Daily As A Maintenance Dose:	800 IU

See Volume II of this series for more on Vitamin E Complex and how to use it to support a healthy cardiovascular system.

---

3 For Vitamin E Complex the author has had the best results with Country Life®, Hauppauge, NY 11788, (800) 645-5768, Puritan's Pride®, Oakdale, NY 11769, (800) 645-1030, Solgar®, Leonia, NJ 07605, (800) 645-2246, and Twinlab®, Ronkonkoma, NY 11779, (800) 645-5626. Puritan's Pride is available by mail order only. The other brands can be purchased at most health foods store and sometimes in the health foods section of supermarkets.

•Reverse Memory Loss

Regaining And Surpassing Your Prior Memory Capacity

1.Take a single dose of Ginkgo Biloba and L-Glutamine three times daily, morning, afternoon, and evening, and continue for four weeks.

2. Reduce to a single dose twice daily, morning and afternoon, and continue as a maintenance dose to help maintain your improved memory and mental function.

Remedy At A Glance (Ginkgo Biloba And L-Glutamine)

Daily For Four Weeks To Relieve Symptoms:	Morning	Afternoon	Evening
	Single Dose	Single Dose	Single Dose
Daily As A Maintenance Dose:	Single Dose	Single Dose	

Notes√√

√ Improvement in memory and other cognitive skills can be noticed within forty-eight hours. The increased mental abilities can last only as long as you continue the daily remedy.

•Improve Learning Abilities And Fight Mental Fatigue

Increasing Analytical Skills And Ability To Assimilate New Information

1. Take a single dose of Ginkgo Biloba and L-Glutamine twice daily, morning and afternoon, and continue for four weeks.

2. At this point you may discontinue the remedy or continue to take a single dose once a day in the morning, as a maintenance dose to help maintain your improved learning abilities.

Remedy At A Glance (Ginkgo Biloba And L-Glutamine)

	Morning	Afternoon
Daily For Four Weeks To Relieve Symptoms:	Single Dose	Single Dose
Daily As A Maintenance Dose (Optional):	Single Dose	

Notes√√

√ Improvement in memory and other cognitive skills can be noticed within twelve hours. The increased mental abilities can last only as long as you continue the daily remedy.

*　　*　　*

The following is a case study written as a short story about one of countless people who have been helped by this remedy: A kosher deli owner in New York City uses this powerful combination to recover his "super memory" and regain his self-esteem.

"If It's Wrong, It's Free"

When the alarm rings at four-thirty, Moshe is already buttoning his wool sweater. As the front door slams behind him, he hears Rose mutter a curse as she silences the clock's punishing ring. He starts down the tall staircase, his wide shoulders hunched in anticipation of assuming the weight of the day's tasks. *So much to do on Mondays, he thinks*. Rose will sleep for another half-hour before stumbling downstairs, eyes hooded, right arm outstretched like a beggar, reaching for the mug of steaming black coffee he always has ready. He chuckles quietly to himself. After almost forty years of marriage, you learn a thing or two about a person. Outside, Moshe crosses the small walkway separating the two buildings, moving fast at the insistence of the bitter March wind, and enters "Havermeyer's Delicatessen." Turning off the burglar alarm, he reaches for a clean apron from a closet just inside the entrance, shrugging it on over his grey sweater. He makes his way through the service area to check the front for deliveries. His movements are slow, deliberate, prideful, as he carefully removes chairs from table tops and rights them on the polished tiled floor.

He stands on the sidewalk in front, elbows bent, fists resting on hips, casting puzzled glances up and down 53rd Street. The icy wind snaps his apron and ruffles his thinning hair. The intemperate breeze matches a coldness he feels growing inside, one that cannot be measured in just degrees Fahrenheit, for it is absence of light as well as heat. And every day the coldness spreads further, squeezing out more light, letting in more darkness.

It is unusually quiet this morning. After five o'clock and still no newspaper trucks? No delivery trucks? Not even the street cleaning equipment is out. And where is Andy with his fresh vegetables from Hunt's Point Market? Moshe watches a lone Yellow Cab speed by, headed down Broadway. And where is Malik, his order man? It isn't like him to be late. Moshe looks east at the slate grey sky, opening slowly to let in the dawn. The towering buildings obscure most of the sky and allow only a narrow oblong to be viewed.

Something nags incessantly at the back of Moshe's mind, as if one part of his brain is doing things and not telling the other. He shrugs off the feeling and goes inside to start the coffee, grateful to be out of the cold. Tension builds in his shoulders as he moves about the large orderly kitchen. When he cannot find the coffee filters immediately, an inexplicable rush of anger and helplessness overtakes him. He pauses against the stainless-steel counter trying to compose himself. Rose will be down soon. His mind attaches to this thought. It calms him as he reaches for the coffee tin a moment later. Rose. They begin every day over coffee, a shared intimacy with the optimism peculiar to beginnings. Rose will help him sort it out, and it seems that more and more he needs Rose to unwind the confusion that tangles his mind. He scoops coffee into the filter, relishing the robust smell and the sound of the grounds crunching against the red plastic cup. He double checks the settings before sitting down, exhaling deeply, resting his head against the wall, while one arm lingers on the cool steel counter and the comforting aroma of percolating coffee slowly fills the room.

Moshe's mind wanders to thoughts of his mother: Thelma still lives in Israel where both his and Rose's families immigrated in 1958. His mother was such a beautiful woman. He can see her face in front of him now, the way she looked that last evening in Havana, standing by the water in a lavender cotton dress, back lighted by a purple and orange sunset. Small girlish features smiling to mask uncertainty. Dark eyes seeing straight into his soul, responding to his needs before he can ask for help. The sweet memory of her mixes with sudden longing and wells up, burning his chest and the backs of his eyes.

He reaches out to touch her, embrace her, saying, "Don't cry, Mama," when he is startled by a firm hand on his shoulder.

"Moshe, what are you doing down here?" Rose asks, glancing at the coffee pot. "Why are you crying, love?" Concern is etched in her face.

"What am I doing?" Moshe responds, wiping tears from his face with the back of one hand and shrugging her arm away with the other. "What do you think I'm doing? Getting ready to open. What else?"

Rose nods her head, sudden comprehension filling her eyes. She says in a soft voice, "Moshe love, today is Sunday. We're closed."

*   *   *

The train ride downtown from Riverdale left my white silk shell stuck like a second skin to my sweating back, with yellow half-moons under my arms--causing me to curse my antiperspirant first and August in New York second. I should have realized the air-conditioning was out when I saw the empty seats in this car. Directly ahead of me in the next car people were jammed together standing room only. A balding black man in a tan suit was squashed against the plexiglass pane in one of the doors separating the cars, still managing to look smug because he'd chosen the one with air-conditioning. I switched to the East Side Shuttle at Grand Central Station, changed trains again at Times Square, and emerged from the muffled brown of the 50th Street subway station into the orange throb of midtown Manhattan. Crossing Broadway against the light, I weaved around the slowly moving cars and the ConEd crew set up in the middle of the intersection.

Broadway oozed yellow with taxis, and the humid air was

14

punched with intermittent sounds of a jackhammer. The taxi drivers shouted epithets at each other and pedestrians alike, and honking horns punctuated their frustration. Even red lights were honked at in the hope of jarring them to green. On the corner, a construction worker barked into the face of a ranting homeless man. A bicycle messenger running the light almost hit me, but I jumped to the curb spoiling his day. New York was in full screech. I could feel the city's heart beating, feel its hot blood rushing in the air around me, infusing everything with energy. New York was just the right tempo for me. I had often felt that the world around me was moving in slow motion, but in New York I was finally in sync.

I avoided a man shoving a leaflet in my face and opened the door to Havermeyer's, triggering several pleasurable sensations. A sudden blast of frigid air cooled the sweat on my skin. Riding on the air like marauders on a train were the familiar smells of spiced sour pickles, corned beef and hot pastrami, onions, mustard, and assorted fresh baked breads and bagels. My mouth began to water before the door closed. The loud hum of the air-conditioning mingled with voices and the clattering of silverware against dishes to create an atmosphere that promised to absorb my presence without notice or comment.

The deli's decor was crisp black and white, and stainless steel. The sturdy green of plastic palms and the deep blues and golds of travel posters lent the only color to the room. Most of its business came from deliveries to the nearby office buildings on Manhattan's west side, between 48th and 58th Street, bordered by Sixth and Eighth Avenues. But its local popularity and close proximity to the theater district brought enough walk-ins to keep ten tables occupied from seven a.m. to closing time--a little after eight.

Richard and Kim waited at a table just inside the door--the only one in full sunlight. The other tables nurtured comfortably in the shade. They were drinking Heinekens; Kim, directly from the bottle; Richard, in a glass mug. I said hello and complained to Kim. "You picked this table didn't you?" Always in pursuit of a tan, she was one of those people who swiveled her chair every ten minutes to match the sun's rotation and get the most direct rays.

"Sorry, I thought *this* was our table," she drawled, with laughing hazel eyes. She eased her blond hair off one shoulder with a casual movement of her hand. We were the same height, weight, and

15

shoe size--and had the same taste in clothes--though we favored different color schemes because of our unlike complexions, hers eggshell, mine honey. Much of my wardrobe was in her closet and vice versa.

"Only because you get here early and select it every time," I said.

"I don't get here early. It's just that you're always late, so how would you know?" She asked, dipping deeply into her Texas accent.

We continued this trite exchange until Richard interrupted us with a stack of thirty-five millimeter contact sheets. As usual, a camera bag sat on the floor between his feet. Tall, olive-complected, and dancer thin, Richard could resolve no mystery he hadn't contemplated through a camera lens. He wore his oak-brown hair long, red beard cut close, and always carried a laugh in his pocket.

I pulled my art layouts from the portfolio and gave them to Richard, showing him where I wanted the photos placed throughout Kim's copy. With the three of us working at our homes and meeting twice a week at Havermeyer's, we'd kept Appletree Productions afloat for five years. The money we earned from Appletree combined with our regular incomes from Hearst Publishing gave us good incomes.

Kim and Richard began to talk about column width and my attention drifted. I watched Malik wrestle with the square neon sign--"If It's Wrong, It's Free"--that hung in the window opposite us. Rose was standing nearby offering directions that Malik ignored. She was a small trim woman with a bubbly, sometimes feisty personality, and short, black curly hair parted long down the middle. I always imagined she is how Betty Boop would have looked at sixty-something.

Moshe came out of the kitchen with an order, shooting Rose a fuming look of disapproval--all the outrage he was capable of.

Malik removed the sign from the two chains supporting it and carried it, under Rose's watchful eye, through the swinging door to the kitchen. He looked me over as he passed and said, "How you doing today my fine sister?" I smiled, but didn't hold the eye contact. Malik was dark-skinned and medium built, with a shaved head and intelligent obsidian eyes. He wore a dashiki under his apron and wire glasses that made him look studious, which was casting to type because he was working on a Masters in anthropology. He gave Kim a quick once over too, nodded, and winked. Without thinking, she moved her left hand to

16

cover the vertical scar on the outside of her right arm. It was a subtle, protective gesture, generated partly by embarrassment and partly because she wasn't used to it being there yet.

Why take down the sign? I'd heard it had been up since the Deli opened twenty-five years ago. It represented the guarantee that if Moshe took your order and made a mistake, everything you ordered was on the house. He took most of the orders and never wrote anything down. And no matter how complicated the order, he never forgot a thing. Newcomers ordered more than they wanted, or could eat, trying to trip him up. Moshe's memory had always been good for business.

His somber presence loomed over us then as Moshe stood patiently, pencil poised over pad, waiting for our orders. In the years I'd been coming to the Deli, I couldn't remember ever seeing him smile. His sad eyes were grey storm clouds, set deep in a soft round face the color of aged porcelain, atop a dense wrestler's body. If anyone could be said to look dependable, it was Moshe. Richard and Kim ordered two more beers and corned beef sandwiches on rye with extra mustard--no onions. My taste was for lemonade, tuna salad with lettuce and tomato on whole wheat toast. Cheesecake was dessert all around.

"You're writing the order, Moshe?" I asked in a loud voice, without thinking. A pained expression came into his already melancholy eyes, and I was sorry immediately. It wasn't the first time my mouth had beaten my brain to the starting gate.

He shrugged. "Sometimes these things happen to a person. I 'hain't complainin'."

*   *   *

Rose pulled the iron gating across the front of the Deli and locked it. She went inside, secured the front door, and switched off the lights as she passed through the service area. She stopped in the small office and turned on the answering machine. At the side door, she opened the closet and put her dirty apron in the hamper. She turned on the burglar alarm before going outside. She was bone tired.

Moshe hadn't spoken to her since she took down the sign. What else could she do? They would be feeding all of Manhattan for nothing if they didn't stop with that promise. Her husband didn't understand what was happening to him. But Rose did. She had seen her own father

17

drift into that fog and never return. She had always been his favorite, then one day he was gone. He simply forgot her, wanted only Jaime, would dismiss her with a wave of one hand when she tried to approach him. He didn't know he was going away, so he didn't have a chance to say goodbye.

She couldn't let that happen to Moshe. Now that she'd discovered there was a choice, they could fight back.

Inside their roomy apartment upstairs, Rose found Moshe sitting in their darkened bedroom on the side of the bed, lost again inside his mind. She sat down beside him and leaned her head on his strong shoulder. She had always felt safe, protected, with her husband by her side. She heard a far off siren and the nearby sounds of traffic going by out front. "My Moshe," she said, and patted his arm gently. He reached one hand up to touch hers. Tears crept down her cheeks, slowly, tiredly, moving with the same despair she felt. Memories, if you let them, can tell you the truth of who and where you are in life. Without honest memories, a person can't really exist here and now. They inhabit another universe, live in a different city, speak an unknown language to unseen souls.

"Don't cry, Rosie," Moshe said, his voice barely audible. "Everything will be all right." He patted her hand, gently covering it with his own.

*   *   *

Havermeyer's was crowded when I entered. Kim waited for me at a table in the rear; Richard was on a photo shoot. The heat wave was over, and Indian summer was coddling the city, turning the leaves in Central Park a dull red.

It had been six weeks since Moshe decided to try Ginkgo Biloba and L-Glutamine. He had resisted when Rose approached him with the idea, denied anything was wrong, and resisted some more. I don't know what he and Rose talked about when I left, but the outline of the little pillbox she gave him the next day was always visible in his apron pocket. Six weeks later the sign went back up. Moshe was ready after four weeks, but it took him another two to summon the courage to put down his order pad.

I watched him strut over to accost the table next to ours--rank newcomers--with a loud recitation of the entire contents of the chalkboard menu, from memory. "...with your choice of strawberry or chocolate chip cheesecake," he finished. The four people at the table, three men and a woman, randomly called out their orders, trying to confuse him. He motioned with the curled fingers of both hands, urging them on. His head was cocked to one side, eyes twinkling. He was almost smiling. The woman asked him if he wanted to write down the orders. He looked over his shoulder to wink at Kim and me. To her he said, "So who needs pencil and paper to remember a few simple items? Besides, what do you care? If it's wrong, it's free."

L-CYSTEINE AND VITAMIN C COMPLEX
Taken Together In Combination

•Heal And Prevent Asthma And Bronchitis
Stopping An Asthma Attack Or Other Serious Breathing Problems
Healing Chronic Asthma, Bronchitis, Nagging Cough, Or Other Respiratory Problems
Preventing Exercise Induced Asthma

•Treat *Any* Temporary Respiratory Illness
Healing A Respiratory Ailment Brought On By Cold, Flu, Or Other Causes

•Guard Against Cigarette Smoker's Damage
Protecting Your Health If You Smoke

•Prevent Or Lessen The Severity Of Hangovers
Taking Steps To Avoid A Hangover *Before* You Have A Drink
Avoiding A Hangover If You Drank Too Much But Haven't Gone To Sleep Yet
Getting Rid Of A Hangover *The Morning After*

•Safeguard Your Body Against Environmental And Other Toxins

Preventing And Slowing Down The Accumulation Of Liver/Age Spots
Protecting Your Health If You Are Regularly Exposed To Second-Hand Smoke, Drugs, Chemicals, Or Pollutants

L-Cysteine is an amino acid, one of the "building blocks" of protein. Vitamin C Complex contains Vitamin C combined with Rutin, Citrus Bioflavinoids, Hesperidin, and sometimes Acerola. When taken together, this combination can have an extraordinary ability to heal and protect lung tissue and promote healthy respiratory function. It can also dramatically lessen the harmful effects of cigarette smoke.

L-Cysteine and Vitamin C Complex can speed up the body's ability to detoxify, especially through the lungs and liver--thereby preventing many harmful effects of environmental toxins, as well as drugs and other chemicals you may ingest. Due to its ability to quickly flush toxins from the liver, the combination can help protect your body from alcohol related damage, preventing hangovers the night before, or greatly relieving them the morning after. It can also be very effective in preventing the formation of brown freckles called liver/age spots, which are essentially a result of years of wear and tear on the liver.

22

Recommended Strength[4]

L-Cysteine--500 mg

Vitamin C Complex--1000 mg (The dosage strength is for Vitamin C only; the other trace components will be present in varying amounts depending upon the brand. You may use Vitamin C alone, without the other trace elements, if you cannot find Vitamin C Complex.)

Recommended Form

L-Cysteine--tablets or capsules

Vitamin C Complex--tablets or capsules

Taken How

A Single Dose: 1 L-Cysteine and 1 Vitamin C Complex (500 mg L-Cysteine, and 1000 mg Vitamin C Complex) taken *together*, with eight ounces of juice or other liquids as directed.

A Double Dose: 2 L-Cysteine and 2 Vitamin C Complex (1000

---

4 For L-Cysteine the author has had the best results with Country Life®, Hauppauge, NY 11788, (800) 645-5768; Puritan's Pride®, Oakdale, NY 11769, (800) 654-1030; and Solgar®, Leonia, NJ 07605, (800) 645-2246. Puritan's Pride is available by mail order only. The other brands can be purchased at most health foods stores and sometimes in the health foods section of supermarkets. There are too many quality brands of Vitamin C Complex to mention here. Try to purchase a brand that obtains Vitamin C and other trace elements from rose hips or other food sources. Try to avoid brands that obtain Vitamin C from synthetic ascorbic acid.

mg L-Cysteine, and 2000 mg Vitamin C Complex) taken *together*, with eight ounces of juice or other liquids as directed.

Side Effects

None observed with either supplement when taken as directed.

Notes√√

√ Taken alone, these supplements will not have the desired therapeutic effect. They should be taken together--at the same time--to be effective as a remedy.

√ The amount of Vitamin C Complex should always equal twice that of L-Cysteine.

•Heal And Prevent Asthma And Bronchitis

Stopping An Asthma Attack Or Other Serious Breathing Problems

1. Take a double dose of L-Cysteine and Vitamin C Complex at the onset.

2. Repeat the double dose every half hour until you have taken a total of four double doses in a ninety minute period, i.e., first double dose at 10:00, then 10:30, 11:00, and 11:30. It can take as little as thirty minutes to lessen your respiratory discomfort. It is recommended that you take all four double doses, even if you feel better before you have completed the entire sequence.

3. Wait a half hour after your last double dose. It is now two hours since you took the first double dose. If you are still feeling discomfort, take a single dose every hour for up to eight hours. Stop when normal breathing returns.

4. If you still experience breathing problems the next day, repeat the procedure as often as necessary to bring relief.

5. When normal breathing returns, it is recommended that you follow the daily regimen below for healing and preventing chronic asthma and bronchitis.

Remedy At A Glance (L-Cysteine And Vitamin C Complex)

	At Start Of Attack	Every Half Hour For 90 Minutes	Every Hour For Up To 8 Hours
To Relieve Asthma Attack:	Double Dose	Double Dose	Single Dose

Notes√√

√ L-Cysteine and Vitamin C Complex should *not* be relied on alone to stop a serious asthma attack, though it can help bring great relief. You should have appropriate medication available to use when any breathing difficulty occurs. The combination is best used as a preventive measure to strengthen and heal the respiratory system and prevent future attacks.

Healing Chronic Asthma, Bronchitis, Nagging Cough, Or Other Respiratory Problems

1. Take a double dose of L-Cysteine and Vitamin C Complex four times daily, i.e., 8:00 a.m., noon, 4:00 p.m., and 8:00 p.m., and continue until your symptoms are gone.

2. Reduce to a double dose three times daily, morning, afternoon, and evening, and continue for four weeks.

3. Continue to take a double dose twice daily, morning and evening, as a maintenance dose to strengthen your respiratory system, *whether or not you are experiencing symptoms.*

Remedy At A Glance (L-Cysteine And Vitamin C Complex)

	8:00 am	Noon	4:00 pm	8:00 pm
Daily To Relieve Symptoms	Double Dose	Double Dose	Double Dose	Double Dose
	Morning	Afternoon	Evening	
Daily For Four Weeks After You Are Better:	Double Dose	Double Dose	Double Dose	
Daily As A Maintenance Dose:	Double Dose		Double Dose	

Notes√√

√ To help heal a chronic respiratory disorder such as asthma, bronchitis, or nagging cough, it is recommended that you also take **Beta Carotene** and **Lecithin**. Beta Carotene accelerates healing anywhere in the body, and Lecithin breaks up mucous to relieve congestion.

Beta Carotene: Use in 25,000 IU softgels only. Take it once a day with your largest meal as directed, regardless of the amount you are taking.

1. Take 250,000 IU (10 softgels) daily for the first two days of each week, i.e., Sunday and Monday.

2. Reduce to 200,000 IU (8 softgels) daily for the next three days, i.e., Tuesday, Wednesday, and Thursday.

3. Reduce to 150,000 IU (6 softgels) daily for the last two days, i.e., Friday and Saturday.

4. Follow this weekly schedule as long as you have any respiratory discomfort, then reduce to 100,000 IU (4 softgels) daily, and continue for four weeks.

5. Continue to take 75,000 (3 softgels) daily, as a maintenance dose to help keep your respiratory system healthy.

26

Remedy At A Glance (Beta Carotene)

	Once A Day With Largest Meal		
	Days 1-2	Days 3-5	Days 6-7
Daily To Relieve Symptoms:	250,000 IU	200,000 IU	150,000 IU
Daily For Four Weeks After You Are Better:	100,000 IU		
Daily As A Maintenance Dose:	75,000 IU		

See Chapter 5 for more on Beta Carotene and how to use it as a remedy to shorten healing time by more than half, and *drastically* reduce wound tenderness and scarring.

Lecithin: Use in 1200 mg softgels only. Take it with eight ounces of juice or other liquids as directed. (Chapter 9 tells you how to use the granular form to supplement your daily doses.)

1. Take 6000 mg (5 softgels) three times daily, morning, afternoon, and evening, and continue as long as you have any respiratory congestion.

2. When your symptoms are gone, reduce to 6000 mg (5 softgels) twice daily, morning and evening, and continue for four weeks.

3. Continue to take 4800 mg (4 softgels) twice daily, morning and evening, as a maintenance dose to help keep your respiratory system free of congestion.

Remedy At A Glance (Lecithin)

	Morning	Afternoon	Evening
Daily To Relieve Congestion:	6000 mg	6000 mg	6000 mg
Daily For Four Weeks: After You Are Better:	6000 mg		6000 mg
Daily As A Maintenance Dose:	4800 mg		4800 mg

See Chapter 9 for more on Lecithin and how to use it to help heal arthritis, prevent bloodclot stroke, lower cholesterol, clean out blocked arteries and heart valves without surgery, prevent arteriosclerosis, end gout, and dissolve gallstones.

Preventing Exercise Induced Asthma

1. Take a double dose of L-Cysteine and Vitamin C Complex one hour before exercising.

2. Take a double dose a half hour before exercising.

3. Take a double dose half way through the workout.

4. Take a double dose directly after the workout.

5. If you still experience breathing problems or other discomfort after exercising, follow the directions above for treating an asthma attack.

Remedy At A Glance (L-Cysteine And Vitamin C Complex)

To Relieve Symptoms:

One Hour Before Exercising	A Half Hour Before	Half Way Through	Directly After
Double Dose	Double Dose	Double Dose	Double Dose

•Treat *Any* Temporary Respiratory Illness

Healing A Respiratory Ailment Brought On By Cold, Flu, Or Other Causes

1. Take a double dose of L-Cysteine and Vitamin C Complex first thing each morning, i.e., 8:00 a.m.

2. Take a single dose one hour later, i.e., 9:00 a.m.

3. Take a double dose every four hours until you have taken three double doses, i.e., 1:00 p.m., 5:00 p.m., and 9:00 p.m.

4. Continue this daily schedule until your symptoms are gone.

5. Reduce to a single dose three times daily, morning, afternoon, and evening, and continue for three days.

6. At this point you may discontinue L-Cysteine and Vitamin C Complex or continue to take a single dose twice daily, morning and evening, as a maintenance dose to help keep your respiratory system healthy.

Remedy At A Glance (L-Cysteine And Vitamin C Complex)

	8:00 am	9:00 am	1:00 pm	5:00 pm	9:00 pm
Daily To Relieve Symptoms:	Double Dose	Single Dose	Double Dose	Double Dose	Double Dose

	Morning	Afternoon	Evening
Daily For Three Days After You Are Better:	Single Dose	Single Dose	Single Dose
Daily As A Maintenance Dose: (Optional)	Single Dose		Single Dose

Notes√√

√ To help heal any respiratory ailment, it is recommended that you also take **Beta Carotene** and **Lecithin**. Beta Carotene accelerates healing anywhere in the body, and Lecithin breaks up mucous to relieve congestion.

Beta Carotene: Use in 25,000 IU softgels only. Take it once a day with your largest meal as directed, regardless of the amount you are taking.

1. Take 250,000 IU (10 softgels) daily, beginning on the first day of your ailment, and continue for up to five days.

2. If you still have symptoms after the fifth day, reduce to 200,000 IU (8 softgels) daily, and continue until your symptoms are gone.

3. Reduce to 100,000 IU (4 softgels) daily, and continue for three days.

4. At this point you may discontinue Beta Carotene or continue to take 50,000 IU (2 softgels) daily, as a maintenance dose to help keep your respiratory system healthy.

Remedy At A Glance (Beta Carotene)

	Once A Day With Largest Meal
Daily For First Five Days To Relieve Symptoms:	250,000 IU
Daily After Fifth Day To Relieve Symptoms:	200,000 IU
Daily For Three Days After You Are Better:	100,000 IU
Daily As A Maintenance Dose: (Optional)	50,000 IU

See Chapter 5 for more on Beta Carotene and how to use it as a remedy to shorten healing time by more than half, and *drastically* reduce wound tenderness and scarring.

Lecithin: Use in 1200 mg softgels only. Take it with eight ounces of juice or other liquids as directed. (Chapter 9 tells you how to use the granular form to supplement your daily doses.)

1. Take 6000 mg (5 softgels) three times daily, morning, afternoon, and evening, and continue as long as you have any respiratory congestion.

2. When your symptoms are gone, reduce to 6000 mg (5 softgels) twice daily, morning and evening, and continue for three days.

3. At this point you may discontinue Lecithin or continue to take 4800 mg (4 softgels) twice daily, morning and evening, as a maintenance dose to help keep your respiratory system free of congestion.

Remedy At A Glance (Lecithin)

	Morning	Afternoon	Evening
Daily To Relieve Congestion:	6000 mg	6000 mg	6000 mg
Daily For Three Days After You Are Better:	6000 mg		6000 mg
Daily As A Maintenance Dose: (Optional)	4800 mg		4800 mg

See Chapter 9 for more on Lecithin and how to use it to help heal arthritis, prevent bloodclot stroke, lower cholesterol, clean out blocked arteries and heart valves without surgery, prevent arteriosclerosis, end gout, and dissolve gallstones.

•Guard Against Cigarette Smoker's Damage

Protecting Your Health If You Smoke

1. Take a double dose of L-Cysteine and Vitamin C Complex three times daily, morning, afternoon, and evening, and continue as a maintenance dose as long as you smoke, to help protect your lungs and other organs from many of the damaging effects.

Remedy At A Glance (L-Cysteine And Vitamin C Complex)

	Morning	Afternoon	Evening
Daily As A Maintenance Dose:	Double Dose	Double Dose	Double Dose

•Prevent Or Lessen The Severity Of Hangovers[5]

Caution: Please do *not* try to use this remedy as a way to drink and drive. Always drink responsibly and designate another driver who does not drink alcohol to get you home safely.

Taking Steps To Avoid A Hangover *Before* You Have A Drink

1. Take a double dose of L-Cysteine and Vitamin C Complex fifteen to thirty minutes before your first drink. Take it with eight ounces of juice or other liquids, but not alcohol.

2. Take a double dose about midway through the event.

---

5 Alcohol destroys Rutin and Vitamin C. If you drink heavily, you can notice tiny, spidery, red and navy lines on your nose, cheeks, and chin, which are ruptured facial capillaries. See Chapter 10 for more on Rutin and how to use it to help prevent arterial ruptures anywhere in the body.

3. Take a double dose fifteen to thirty minutes before bedtime.

4. Take a double dose as soon as you wake up.

5. If you still experience symptoms of a hangover, take a single dose every hour until all symptoms are gone.

Remedy At A Glance (L-Cysteine And Vitamin C Complex)

To Help Prevent Hangovers:

15-30 Minute Before You Drink	Midway	15-30 Minutes Before Bed	Upon Awakening	Hourly If You Still Have Symptoms
Double Dose	Double Dose	Double Dose	Double Dose	Single Dose

Notes√√

√ It is recommended that you also take **Vitamin B12** to help you wake up faster and feel alert, without the clouded thinking and sluggish reactions usually associated with a hangover.

Vitamin B12: Use in 1000 mcg tablets, capsules, or sublingual form. Take it with eight ounces of juice or other liquids as directed, but not alcohol. (Sublingual form is dissolved under the tongue and requires no liquids.)

1. Take 1000 mcg fifteen to thirty minutes before you have a drink.

2. Take 2000 mcg *directly* before you go to sleep.

3. Take 1000 mcg as soon as you wake up.

33

Remedy At A Glance (Vitamin B12)

	15-30 Minutes Before You Drink	Directly Before Bed	Upon Awakening
To Help Prevent Hangovers:	1000 mcg	2000 mcg	1000 mcg

See Chapter 11 for more on Vitamin B12 and how to us it as a remedy to help prevent fatigue and stop tingling extremities.

Avoiding A Hangover If You Drank Too Much But Haven't Gone To Sleep Yet

1. Take a double dose of L-Cysteine and Vitamin C Complex--as soon as you can--with eight ounces of juice or other liquids, but not alcohol.

2. Take a double dose a half hour later.

3. Take a double dose an hour after that.

4. Take a double dose as soon as you awaken, whether or not you have a hangover.

5. If you still experience symptoms of a hangover, take a single dose every hour until all symptoms are gone.

Remedy At A Glance (L-Cysteine And Vitamin C Complex)

To Help Prevent Hangovers:

First Dose	Half Hour Later	One Hour Later	Upon Awakening	Hourly If You Still Have Symptoms
Double Dose	Double Dose	Double Dose	Double Dose	Single Dose

Notes√√

√ It is recommended that you also take **Vitamin B12** to help you wake up faster and feel alert, without the clouded thinking and sluggish reactions usually associated with a hangover.

Vitamin B12: Use in 1000 mcg tablets, capsules, or sublingual form. Take it with eight ounces of juice or other liquids, but not alcohol. (Sublingual form is dissolved under the tongue and requires no liquids.)

1. Take 2000 mcg *directly* before you go to sleep.

2. Take 2000 mcg as soon as you wake up.

Remedy At A Glance (Vitamin B12)

	Directly Before Bed	Upon Awakening
To Help Prevent Hangovers:	2000 mcg	2000 mcg

See Chapter 11 for more on Vitamin B12 and how to use it as a remedy to help prevent fatigue and stop tingling extremities.

Getting Rid Of A Hangover *The Morning After*

1. Take a double dose of L-Cysteine and Vitamin C Complex as soon as you wake up. Take it with eight ounces of juice or other liquids, but not alcohol.

2. Take a double dose a half hour later.

3. Take a single dose every hour until all symptoms are gone.

Remedy At A Glance (L-Cysteine And Vitamin C Complex)

	Upon Awakening	Half Hour Later	Hourly Until Symptoms Are Gone
To Get Rid Of Hangovers:	Double Dose	Double Dose	Single Dose

Notes√√

√ It is recommended that you also take **Vitamin B12** to help you wake up faster and feel alert, without the clouded thinking and sluggish reactions usually associated with a hangover.

Vitamin B12: Use in 1000 mcg tablets, capsules, or sublingual form. Take it with eight ounces of juice or other liquids, but not alcohol. (Sublingual form is dissolved under the tongue and requires no liquids.)

1. Take 2000 mcg as soon as you wake up.

2. Take 2000 mcg two hours later.

Remedy At A Glance (Vitamin B12)

	Upon Awakening	Two Hours Later
To Get Rid Of Hangovers:	2000 mcg	2000 mcg

See Chapter 11 for more on Vitamin B12 and how to use it to help prevent fatigue and stop tingling extremities.

•Safeguard Your Body Against Environmental And Other Toxins

Preventing And Slowing Down The Accumulation Of Liver/Age Spots

1. Take a double dose of L-Cysteine and Vitamin C Complex three times daily, morning, afternoon, and evening, and continue for six weeks.

2. Reduce to a single dose three times daily, morning, afternoon, and evening, and continue for six weeks.

3. Reduce to a single dose twice daily, morning and evening, and continue as a maintenance dose to help prevent liver/age spots.

Remedy At A Glance (L-Cysteine And Vitamin C Complex)

	Morning	Afternoon	Evening
Daily For Six Weeks To Relieve Symptoms:	Double Dose	Double Dose	Double Dose
Daily For Six Weeks To Relieve Symptoms:	Single Dose	Single Dose	Single Dose
Daily As A Maintenance Dose:	Single Dose		Single Dose

Notes√√

√ If you already have liver spots, you will need to use a bleaching creme regularly in order to erase them, but you *can* bleach them out. And with daily use, L-Cysteine and Vitamin C Complex can prevent new ones from forming, or considerably slow down their accumulation.

Protecting Your Health If You Are Regularly Exposed To Second-Hand Smoke, Drugs, Chemicals, Or Pollutants

1. Take a single dose of L-Cysteine and Vitamin C Complex twice daily, morning and evening, and continue as a maintenance dose to help protect your health from toxins.

2. If you feel you have already been exposed to significant levels of toxins, follow the twelve week regimen above, under age/liver spots, before you reduce to the maintenance dose recommended here.

Remedy At A Glance (L-Cysteine And Vitamin C Complex)

	Morning	Evening
Daily As A Maintenance Dose:	Single Dose	Single Dose

*   *   *

The following is a case study written as a short story about one of countless people who have been helped by this remedy: A divorced dad kidnaps his children and flees from Dallas to Mexico, where he learns to fight his own rash temperament while using this combination to overcome asthma.

"Me And Henry"

My dad said it's not possible for a father to kidnap his own children. That children belong to both parents for always, no matter what the 'jadishal system says about custody. Before my parents got divorced, seems like they never stopped arguing. After it, they just stopped talking. They disagreed so much that I think they wanted it that way. Otherwise, how could they always not agree on anything? Like with ice cream. Mama said we couldn't eat dessert during the week, only on weekends, in the afternoon, after we ate some *real* food. Daddy said ice cream was *real* food and snuck it to us every chance he got, sometimes right before supper on the days he picked us up after school. It never ruined my appetite, just Henry's.

They even disagreed on how to get divorced: At night when she thought we were asleep, Mama said, "You need to get counseling, Arthur, while there's still a chance for us." But my dad refused. "There's nothing wrong with me," he said. Me and Henry couldn't understand everything we heard, because we were only nine and six. But we knew Daddy had done something real bad--didn't know what, but real bad--that made Mama so angry she couldn't find her way back to where she wasn't mad anymore. I know there's still a place in her heart for him. I can see it in her eyes when she doesn't notice I'm there. She'll put down the newspaper, stop chopping the onions, pause with fingers above the computer keyboard, when a memory taps her shoulder. I know she's thinking about him. She's looking past the ugly words and mean acts to that place where she still loves him, but she's lost the directions there.

After the divorce, me and Henry were home with Mama in Highland Park during the week, for school and scouts and music lessons. Friday nights to Sunday afternoons we spent with Daddy in his loft near downtown, playing video games, eating fast food, and watching movies. He ran a computer consultancy business out of the

38

front of the loft, and lived in the back in a two-bedroom apartment with a far off view of I-35. Daddy didn't have many rules for when we visited; he didn't make us do homework. (We did it anyway because Mama wouldn't let us play when we got home on Sundays until it was done.) We went to bed when we felt like it, ate whatever we pleased. His only two rules: no gum chewing and no fighting.

The last time Daddy picked us up at aftercare he was late. There was just me and Henry left in the basement playroom. He leaned over to peek below the wall before he reached the bottom of the wooden staircase. His eyes were sorry, and I knew right away he was keeping a secret. He apologized for being late and, hunching down like a gorilla, chased us around the room grunting and hooting and scratching until we were weak with laughter, squealing in delight, and gasping for breath on the floor. We lay there still sprouting giggles, sprawled between the green plastic slide and the Dr. Pepper soda machine, with my dad's breathing making a kind of in-out melody as he wheezed, trying to squeeze more air out of each breath. He was really cool about his asthma, no matter how bad it got. I watched as he leaned back on one elbow and took an inhaler from his jacket pocket, quickly pumping and inhaling twice. I forgot to hold my breath, and I could taste the bitter mist on the back of my tongue.

We grabbed our backpacks and followed him up stairs, racing ahead, cutting across the empty playground. As soon as he unlocked the van we piled in. Friday nights with our dad were always the same: Pizza Hut, Boll Weevil, or KFC for dinner, except on special occasions when we went to Black Angus, then Baskin-Robbins for dessert. On the way to the loft we rented videos.

But after dinner on this Friday our dad said he had a surprise. We were going to take a drive. Where was a secret.

Henry fell asleep on the rear seat as soon as he finished his ice cream and licked his fingers. He was lying on his side with his head resting on a folded arm. His other hand was tucked between his knees. Pistachio and chocolate smeared the corners of his mouth. From the front seat next to my dad I watched other cars go by, counting how many had children. There weren't any jazz tapes playing, adding to the air of expectancy, and leaving only the sound of the tires spinning against the road. I closed my eyes on the sad whine. When I opened them again it was almost dark. The sooty towers of an oil refinery whizzed by on my side, outlined by a tangerine-colored sky. I remembered what my teacher, Mrs. Avila, told us about the four directions: If the sun was setting on my side of the car, we were headed south. Toward Mexico.

"How come we're going so far in this direction?" I asked. "This is way past our exit. We only go this far when visiting Nanna, but she lives in Dallas now."

My dad turned his head and studied my face but didn't answer. Instead, he took an inhaler out of his pocket, and pumped-and-inhaled. I remembered to hold my breath. He took the inhaler out of his mouth and shook it next to his right ear. Then he capped it and returned it to his pocket with a long frustrated sigh. A minute later he remembered the one in the glove compartment and reached across me to get it. I forgot to hold my breath as he removed the cap for two quick pumps-and-inhale, a deep breath, and another pump-and-inhale. The vapors smelled like the back end of a drugstore and made me want to spit. He replaced the cap and put the inhaler in his pocket, putting the near-empty one in the glove compartment.

"Where are we going, Daddy?" I prodded, a little worried now, remembering things he'd said about not getting to see me and Henry enough. Our mom's a lawyer, and Daddy said she 'nipulated the system to get everything she wanted in the divorce. He turned to look at me again, not looking so sure of himself now, then moved his eyes back to the road. As I watched him, the lights from oncoming traffic highlighted his handsome brown face an instant at a time, then withdrew, dropping it suddenly back into shadow.

*   *   *

Monica was always telling him he was crazy. Now he'd gone and proved his wife wasn't lying by abducting his own kids. Arthur thought this as he held his last inhaler close to his right ear and shook it, judging he had enough inhalant to last until he crossed the border. His prescription had expired, but he would have no problem refilling it in Mexico.

Monica was a good wife and mother. Too good. Maybe that was part of his problem. Her excellence made his own haplessness so much more evident. He tried to explain this to her once after they made love. Lying close in the dark it was easier to say. She misunderstood his reason for sharing, didn't know that he wasn't seeking reassurance, which she had given him aplenty, listing all the reasons he shouldn't feel the way he felt. When what he wanted to know was how she managed to never feel that way. Never doubt, second guess, waver, or fret.

Just after midnight on Saturday morning, with a full moon relishing its reign, Arthur pulled off I-35 into the parking lot of Motel 6, south of San Antonio, about a hundred twenty five miles from the New Laredo border crossing. He planned to cross into Mexico tomorrow around noon--had to get the kids up, washed, dressed, fed, and stopped from fighting. Then south to Monterrey for an overnight stay. Sunday morning he would venture deeper into Mexico to the Port of Tampico, where his cousin Ted and wife Yuki would be waiting. From there a boat would take the Johnsons to Merida by way of Progresso.

Arthur watched his children sleeping in the queen bed next to the window. He had used one of Monica's credit cards to pay for the room, long since having ruined his own credit. A dirty trick to stick his wife with the wages of his escapade; she wouldn't be happy. When she was angry Monica expressed herself in broad caustic strokes. She was capable of a dark, destructive wrath, but he knew she'd never cancel the card as long as he had the kids. First, to make sure he could buy whatever he needed for them. Second, so she could trace the receipts, find him, and take the kids back. He congratulated himself for being smart enough to get a large cash advance in San Antonio, immediately converting it to American Express traveler's checks.

He had prepared a story for his children, *his* children, but when his daughter, Terry, asked him pointedly where they were going, asked in that way of saying she already knew the answer, like her mother, he couldn't bring himself to lie. Without Monica around, he would be their only role model. If he lied, they would find out in a matter of days. That left the truth, which he wasn't capable of just yet. Maybe Monica had nothing to worry about, but it occurred to him then that he might.

*　　　*　　　*

At first I missed the tap-tap-tap, sounding so much like a bird

41

in a tree that it was lost in the tlack-tlack-tlack of my old Brother typewriter. I was in the bedroom using a glass-topped dressing table as a work area, because that room had the only ceiling fan in the house. The beaten fan hung loosely, and I worried that it would rip lose one day and whirl around the room, slicing everything in its way; but that didn't stop me from having it on day and night.

I turned off the radio, playing an old Jose Jose love song, left the bedroom and walked eight feet to my front door to investigate. I didn't open it because I could see through the glass-louvers no one was there. Then it came again, stronger. Tap-tap-tap. I looked out back on the small patio. No one. Again I heard the tapping. I returned to the bedroom and followed the sound into the bathroom.

I called, "Hello?"

"Hello," came the flat response. A child. American.

"Where are you?" I asked.

"Down here," she said, as though it should be obvious to me where she was.

I kicked off my sandals and stood barefoot on the toilet bowl to reach the small screenless window and look out. Two feet below looking up at me was a young girl about ten. She had chocolate brown skin, pretty features in a narrow face, and two neat braids that hung to her shoulder, each closed with a red-ribbon bow. She was barefoot, dressed in white shorts, and a black and red Bulls tee-shirt. She had been knocking on my bathroom wall with a small rock as if it were a door that could be opened.

"Do you know how to light a gas oven?" She asked.

I glanced at the blue and white box of wooden matches she was holding. "A gas oven? Where's Yuki?"

"Excuse my manners. My name's Terry Johnson. Me and my brother Henry and our dad came down here to live with Aunt Yuki and Uncle Ted for a while," she said, rolling her words out, emphasizing her accent. "And now me and Henry, we want to heat up a cheese quesadilla casserole, but the oven won't turn on by itself." A slight whuff of gas floated by on the muggy air.

"Isn't anyone at home with you?"

"Uncle Ted's playing in an afternoon away game. He's with the Mexican Baseball League," she said, sounding proud. "Aunt Yuki's dropping him off, and then she's going to take my dad to the University

Sell your books at sellbackyourBook.com!

Go to sellbackyourBook.com
and get an instant price quote.
We even pay the shipping - see
what your old books are worth
today!

Inspected By:maria_qc

0007147 8330

to pick up an application. He's trying to get a job teaching English to people taking tests to be pilots and traffic controllers."

"Oh, your father's a teacher."

"No."

I thought for a second before saying, "Ahh, I think you should wait for Yuki to get back. The ball park and the University are both just ten minutes away. I'm sure she'll be home soon." I didn't want to get sucked into being a substitute adult for a neighbor's child. I had taken a semester off from school to live in Mexico and write a novel. I had no responsibilities except to my work, and I wanted to keep it that way.

"If you don't want to help me, I'm sure I can do it by myself," she said, turning away.

Maybe it was just imagination, but I thought I heard accusation in her tone. Anyway, before she reached the door I caved in. "Hold it," I said. "I'm coming over."

I went out my back door, crossed the cement patio, and opened the gate in the high wooden fence that separated my area from the large common plaza and the other houses in the complex. I was renting a one-bedroom in *Colonia Aleman*, a suburb of Merida, Mexico, thirty minutes by bus and ten by car from the downtown *Zocalo*--the main plaza. Ted and Yuki rented a house behind mine. The owners, the Alcazars, lived in the large main residence on the corner of *Calle* 31 and *Calle* 33. Two other houses were occupied by several medical students enrolled at the University of Merida. The last three cottages sheltered the Alcazars' daughters and their families. Each of our rear patios opened to the common plaza, and the daughters' cottages could only be reached by way of it.

Merida is an orderly Mexican city of approximately one hundred thousand; ninety-five percent of its streets are named with numbers--odd numbers moving on a north/south axis and even numbers going east/west. It is also progressive, boasting museums, an international airport, gourmet and ethnic restaurants, and you can drink the water. As capital of the Yucatan State, political awareness is part of the culture. The people call themselves *Yucatecos!* not Mexicans, and are quick to remind Americans what we owe them: that Mexico had a choice in 1846 between mounting a civil war against them when they tried to secede, or fighting a border war with the United States, who was infringing into the Mexican territories of what are now California,

43

Arizona, New Mexico and Texas. Mexico invested its military resources in keeping together its union, and forfeited millions of acres to us.

I let myself in the gate to the small patio next door and knocked on the door sill. The front door was propped open with a large green-glass Buddha. With my house in front and the avocado trees high overhead, this little place remained unsunned most of the day. It was cool and shadowy inside. The after odor of incense hovered in the air, scenting the disturbing smell of cooking gas. Terry was standing just inside the door still holding the matches. She introduced her brother Henry who was standing next to and slightly behind her. He seemed too old to be getting so much comfort from the thumb stuck in his mouth. He had a round face with fair brown skin, freckles, and short woolly brown hair. His grey shorts and black tee were ironed smooth, just like his sister's clothes. Henry had a sad expression on his face and didn't respond when I spoke to him. Both children were clean and obviously well cared for, but there was something melancholy about them, as though they were weighted down by a common misery.

Ted and Yuki's house was small and furnished with the same type of worn out, mismatched pieces as mine. But Yuki had laid oriental rugs from her native Japan on the bare linoleum and hung colorful tapestries on the walls. There were beaded curtains in all the doorways, and windchimes and plants moved in the breeze at every window. I followed Terry into the kitchen, fitted like mine with retro '50's appliances in a garish aqua color. In the corner of the Formica counter were several prescription bottles and two asthma inhalers. After several failed attempts at lighting Yuki's oven, I took the casserole to my house to heat. I also took the box of matches. I was happy to get out of Yuki's neat kitchen where I felt like an intruder.

As I was returning with the steaming casserole wrapped in one of the Alcazar's bath towels (they were wafer thin so I was moving fast), Yuki pulled into the driveway in her red Volkswagon Beetle. In the passenger seat was a man I assumed was the childrens' father. Easy to see where the kids got at least some of their good looks. He was medium height, wearing a sleeveless white tee shirt, white pants and leather *huaraches*. Henry had his father's fair coloring; apparently Terry got her dark beauty from her mother.

Arthur didn't wait to be introduced. He left Yuki with the bags and swaggered over. We were both genuinely amused when our handshake caused a mutual shock of static electricity; amazing in the humid air. His arms and shoulders were well defined without looking as though he worked hard at keeping them that way. I tried to appear nonchalant, but there was no ignoring the sexual pull of the man. Yuki asked me to stay for lunch and I accepted.

The cheese and bean quesadilla casserole tasted better than it looked and went nicely with the rice and bean-sprout salad Yuki prepared in just minutes. We ate lunch outside and drank tart *limonada* while sitting on pillows, shaded by the glossy leaves on the avocado trees. Above us, birds gossiped and squabbled and sang praises. The Alcazar daughters were making fresh corn tortillas in the outside kitchen; the hot, toasted corn aroma would have made my mouth water if I weren't already eating. The women had the radio tuned loudly to XMER, playing Mexican rock and roll. I caught myself humming along as I ate.

*   *   *

Arthur noticed his breath getting short when he finished eating. He dug deeper and deeper, and the effort rocked his strong body forward and back with each inhalation. He went inside to retrieve an inhaler from the kitchen table, fighting down the slight panic that always nipped him when he couldn't breathe normally. Take it easy. It will never be like it was before, when they hadn't believed he was having that first attack. He was seven, and they had waited almost too long before taking him to the emergency room. His parents, and his grandmother who lived with them, were having a party. Had been drinking all day. It was his sister, only four years older, who finally got through to them. From that time, he used his illness as a means of control--first with his parents, then others.

*   *   *

I found myself taking a deep breath with Arthur every time he tried but couldn't. When I realized what I was doing, I stopped before I could hyperventilate. He must have seen the distress on my face, because he explained that he'd been having a problem with the Mexican

45

medication; said it didn't always work, but he would be fine soon.

"I have something next door that can help your asthma," I offered.

"You have asthma too?" he asked.

"No, but I like to experiment with food supplements. I have a combination that works on asthma and bronchitis."

He nodded and beckoned with the hand holding the inhaler. "I'll try anything," he said.

As we walked back to my house, I gave Arthur the matches and told him how I'd met Terry. He didn't seem concerned.

I loaned him a bottle each of L-Cysteine and Vitamin C Complex and gave him specific instructions on how to take the supplements. I also gave him the phone number of a wholesaler in Tijuana and told him he could pay me back when he received his first order. He took the supplements but didn't use them consistently. His behavior was always the same: the first few days of the week he followed my instructions, felt better, then stopped taking the vitamins and suffered an asthma attack before the weekend. After the attack, he would start taking them again until he felt better. I reminded him it was possible to keep his asthma under control, but only if he stuck to the schedule and took the supplements every day.

One evening about two months later, right after the six o'clock news, Arthur knocked at my front door and asked if we could talk. I didn't have a television, but Senora Alcazar was hearing-impaired and played her set so loudly that everyone for two blocks had to listen to the *noticias* with her. I was grateful the one news half-hour was all she watched. Arthur was wearing a turquoise fishnet tee shirt, jeans, and plenty of Calvin Klein's Obsession. I reminded myself that he was a man with two children, an ex-wife he apparently wasn't over, and lots of unresolved emotional problems. I assumed he wanted to discuss his asthma, but in no time he had called me "sister," and asked me to help him with his childrens' lessons. He said they were being home taught. His voice was low and velvety, the sound of his explanation mixing with the chorus of crickets, cicadas, barking dogs, and other seductive night voices that drifted through the open louvers.

"I can't help you," I said, and the look of surprise that blossomed on his face made me laugh. I apologized and tried to explain why I came to Mexico.

46

Arthur nodded but didn't say anything. He'd been certain I would help him. Evidently he was used to people, or at least women, giving him what he wanted. After a few moments of calculated reflection, he said, "It would be easy, only take an hour or two a day."

I shook my head, and said, "If it's so easy why do you need my help?"

He laughed and looked embarrassed.

Not willing to give him any slack I said, "Besides the actual teaching, I would have to allot time for planning the classes, correcting tests and homework, answering questions about the lessons. I don't have the time, and frankly I don't want the responsibility." Hey, they weren't *my* kids. "How much time are you spending at it now?"

"I haven't actually started their lessons yet," he said, blushing, and looked away.

"But you've been here over two months. What do they do all day while you work?"

He pulled an inhaler out of his pocket, saying, "They play games and read comic books and watch cartoons like other kids."

"You're not taking the supplements regularly," I said, changing the subject.

"How do you know that?" he asked and smiled, shifting closer to me on the sofa. It was such a casual movement I didn't know what it meant, if anything.

"If you were you wouldn't need the inhaler." I tried to keep my voice neutral, but irritability gave it an edge. Arthur knew the supplements worked, so why wasn't he taking them?

When he didn't respond, I shifted the conversation back to his children, asking, "Why did you come down here during the school year without a plan for their education?"

"Now you're starting to sound like my wife," he said and smiled, adding quickly, "Don't worry, that's a compliment." His eyes went all honey and milk at the thought of her. He moved back, opening up the space between us on the sofa.

"I did something stupid I'm not sure how to undo," he ventured.

The wind was whipping itself up outside, slipping in through the louvers, cooling my shoulders. I wasn't sure I wanted to hear Arthur's confession, so I kept my options open by remaining silent. He told his story without prompting from me, and it sounded like a first-telling, like it had been waiting for the right set of ears. By the time he finished, a decision was sitting in his eyes. We chatted for a while longer, but he didn't ask for my opinion afterward, and I didn't offer it.

Over the next eight weeks Arthur tried to become the kind of parent he'd chided his wife for being. Committed. Terry continued to knock on my bathroom wall for impromptu conversations, while I stood on the toilet bowl and she talked with her head resting back on her shoulders. From what Arthur had told me, and from what I could glean from the children's behavior, before this he had been more playmate than parent.

He also got serious about the asthma remedy, taking the supplements at the same time each day. Each week his asthma improved. After six weeks he no longer needed an inhaler as long as he took the supplements three times a day.

*   *   *

I was packing for my return to New York City when I heard a commotion coming from the bathroom. I climbed on the toilet bowl and looked out the window. Arthur and Ted were moving suitcases, cardboard soup boxes, and duffel bags into Arthur's van. Yuki was standing with Henry and Terry talking quietly. When Terry saw me she smiled and came bouncing over. We had shared many conversations through this bathroom window over the past four months.

"You're moving out, Terry?" Before she could answer Henry raced over, shouting, "We're-going-back-home-to-Highland-Park-Dallas-the-best-damn-state-in-the-union-Texas!" That was about ten words more than I'd heard him speak since we met.

Arthur scolded him. "What did I tell you about cussing, Henry?"

Henry turned to his father, indignant, "We didn't have all these rules with you before."

Arthur started to respond but changed his mind and ordered his children into the van. While they gave good-bye hugs to Yuki and Ted, he approached the bathroom window.

"I really appreciate what you did," he said.

"I didn't do anything, remember?"

48

He laughed. "Maybe that's exactly what I needed. But I'm talking about my asthma. Its gone mostly. I owe you for that, and I don't know, ahh...."

"Pass it on. Use the information to help someone else, and the debt to me will be erased."

He nodded and searched the back of my eyes like a man pondering the loss of something he never had. "So, thanks for what you did do," he said in a soft voice. "And what you didn't do."

I exchanged addresses with Yuki and Ted before I left but never bothered to get Arthur's or give him mine. He was on his way back to someone, maybe not a better man, but at least one who might be willing to make an effort to get there. I hope she took him back.

CHAPTER 4

L-LYSINE

•Suppress And Prevent Genital Herpes, Cold Sores, The Flu, And Other Common Viruses

L-Lysine is an amino acid, one of the "building blocks" of protein. Taken as directed it can stop genital herpes, cold sores, the flu, and other common viruses from surviving in your system, actually disrupting the virus's DNA replication cycle.

This is important to know for two reasons:

First, each year we are under attack from new and more deadly strains of flu viruses that claim lives.

Second, it is estimated that approximately one in five Americans carries the herpes virus, which can show up as an outbreak of genital herpes or cold sores. A large number of these people have never had an outbreak and are not aware they have the condition. One reason so many people are carriers is that herpes is part of the same family of diseases experienced in childhood, like chicken pox. If you had one of these childhood diseases, you are probably carrying a herpes virus even if you have never had an outbreak. Unfortunately, if you have a herpes virus you can pass it to another person when you have no symptoms, even if you have *never* had an outbreak. For example, in a recent survey, a third of the participants who caught genital herpes from their infected partners did so when their partners had no symptoms.

The number of individuals with herpes will probably continue to rise, while the high cost and side effects of prescription drugs cause many people to avoid using them. L-Lysine is an alternative treatment that is safe, inexpensive, and gentle on your system. It can work quickly to suppress herpes viruses on the same day as an outbreak. Chronic cases can be prevented by taking a daily maintenance dose and increasing the dosage at the first sign of an outbreak: Your body's warning plus your timely response *can* equal prevention. L-Lysine is so effective that it may someday eliminate the unnecessary stigma attached to herpes, because it is now possible to suppress and prevent the condition easily and naturally.

Recommended Strength[6]

1000 mg

Recommended Form

Tablets or capsules

Taken How

With eight ounces of juice or other liquids as directed.

Side Effects

None observed when taken as directed.

•Suppress And Prevent Genital Herpes, Cold Sores, The Flu, And Other Common Viruses

1.   Take 5000 mg of L-Lysine at the first sign of herpes, the flu, or other virus.

2. Take 5000 mg four times daily, i.e., 8:00 a.m., 1:00 p.m., 6:00 p.m., and 11:00 p.m., and continue until your symptoms are gone.

---

6 For L-Lysine the author has had the best results with Country Life®, Hauppauge, NY 11799, (800) 645-5768; Puritan's Pride®, Oakdale, NY 11769, (800) 645-1030; Solgar®, Leonia, NJ 07605, (800) 645-2246, and Twin Lab®, Ronkonkoma, NY 11779, (800) 645-5626. Puritan's Pride is available by mail order only. The other brands can be purchased at most health foods stores and sometimes in the health foods section of supermarkets.

3. Reduce to 2000 mg three times daily, morning, afternoon, and evening, and continue for three days.

4. If you are treating a herpes virus, it is recommended that you continue to take 2000 mg twice daily, morning and evening, as a maintenance dose to help prevent the condition.

5. If you are treating another virus, at this point you may discontinue L-Lysine or continue to take 1000 mg twice daily, morning and evening, as a maintenance dose to help prevent the condition.

Remedy At A Glance (L-Lysine)

At First Sign Of Herpes Or Other Virus, And Daily To Relieve Symptoms:	8:00 am	1:00 pm	6:00 pm	11:00 pm
	5000 mg	5000 mg	5000 mg	5000 mg
	Morning	Afternoon	Evening	
Daily For Three Days After You Are Better:	2000 mg	2000 mg	2000 mg	
Daily As A Maintenance Dose If Treating Herpes :	2000 mg		2000 mg	
Daily As A Maintenance Dose (Optional)	1000 mg		1000 mg	

Notes√√

√ It cannot be overemphasized that you have to flood your system with L-Lysine in order for it to be effective as a remedy against herpes, flu, or other viruses. It is important to take every dose on time, and not miss a single one. Be aware that taking more than 5000 milligrams at one time can result in short-term diarrhea.

√ If you know you have been exposed to a herpes virus but have never had an outbreak, it is recommended that you take 2000 mg of L-Lysine twice daily, morning and evening, as a maintenance dose to help keep the virus dormant.

53

√ It is common knowledge that herpes viruses are often stress related. If you believe that stress is a cause of your outbreaks, it is recommended that you also take **Kava Kava**, because it can greatly relieve stress and anxiety.

Kava Kava (Piper Methysticum): Use a root extract formula that contains from thirty to fifty-five percent kavalactones.[7] Look for percentages on the label, because formulas vary among manufacturers: a 250 milligram formula may have a higher percentage of kavalactones than a 300 milligram formula. Use softgels or capsules only. Take it with juice or other liquids as directed.

1. Take two softgels or capsules each morning, and one in the early afternoon, and continue as a maintenance dose to help lessen anxiety and stress.

2. Extended daily use of Kava Kava can cause dry, flaky skin and itching. For this reason, it is important not to exceed the recommended daily dosages. If you experience these symptoms, add one tablespoon of extra-virgin olive oil to your daily diet, used directly from the bottle--not in cooking. Wait a few days and see if this alleviates your dry skin. If not, you will have to decrease your daily intake of Kava Kava below that recommended here.

Remedy At A Glance (Kava Kava)

	Morning	Early Afternoon
Daily To Relieve Stress:	2 Softgels or Capsules	1 Softgel or Capsule

7 For Kava Kava, the author has had the best results with <u>Enzymatic Therapy®</u> ("Kava-55"), Green Bay, WI 54311, (800) 783-2286 (en espanol (800) 552-6338); and <u>Solaray®</u>, Park City, UT 84068. Both brands are available at most health foods stores and sometimes in the health foods section of supermarkets.

See Volume II of this series for more on Kava Kava and how to use it as a remedy to fight stress and anxiety.

√ How do you know whether you have the flu or just a cold? Cold symptoms usually occur from the neck up--sore throat, trouble swallowing, headache, sinus problems, sneezing, stuffy and/or runny nose, watery eyes, and low fever. The primary symptoms of the flu are the rapid onset of muscle aches and fatigue. Other flu symptoms can include respiratory inflammation, congestion, runny nose, headache, and high fever. Generally, the flu comes on faster and leaves the person feeling truly exhausted. Colds come on slower and are less debilitating.

√ Many people find additional relief from flu symptoms by also taking the Bee Pollen and Vitamin C Complex cold remedy found in Chapter 7.

√ Certain foods produce mucous in your system and should be avoided or kept to a minimum while treating the flu: (1) all milk products including ice cream, butter, yogurt, whipped cream, sour cream, etc, (2) all sugar products, especially candy and other sweet desserts, (3) alcohol of any kind.

√ Be aware that the symptoms of Lyme disease, a bacterial infection transmitted to people by infected ticks, can mimic those of the flu. (Also, look for one or more red bite spots that increase in size.) If you have flu symptoms and bite marks, and there is any chance you may have contracted Lyme disease, such as having gone on a recent camping trip or walk in a wooded area, you should consult a doctor immediately. L-Lysine is a remedy for *viral* based infections, not those that are *bacterial* based.

√ To help heal the flu, it is recommended that you also take **Beta Carotene, Lecithin**, and **B12**. Beta Carotene accelerates healing anywhere in the body. Lecithin breaks up mucous to relieve congestion, and B12 helps relieve the physical exhaustion that accompanies the flu.

Beta Carotene: Use 25,000 IU softgels only. Take it once a day with your largest meal as directed, regardless of the amount you are taking.

1. Take 250,000 IU (10 softgels) daily, beginning on the first day of the flu, and continue for up to five days.

2. If you still have symptoms after the fifth day, reduce to 200,000 IU (8 softgels) daily, and continue at this level until your symptoms are gone.

3. Reduce to 100,000 IU (4 softgels) daily, and continue for three days.

4. At this point you may discontinue Beta Carotene or continue to take 50,000 IU (2 softgels) daily, as a maintenance dose to help promote good health in bone and soft tissue.

Remedy At A Glance (Beta Carotene)

	Once A Day With Largest Meal
Daily For First Five Days To Relieve Symptoms:	250,000 IU
Daily After Fifth Day To Relieve Symptoms:	200,000 IU
Daily For Three Days After You Are Better:	100,000 IU
Daily As A Maintenance Dose: (Optional)	50,000 IU

See Chapter 5 for more on Beta Carotene and how to use it as a remedy to shorten healing time by more than half, and *drastically* reduce wound tenderness and scarring.

Lecithin: Use in 1200 mg softgels only. Take it with eight ounces of juice or other liquids as directed. (Chapter 9 tells you how to use the granular form to supplement your daily doses.)

1. Take 6000 mg (5 softgels) three times daily, morning, afternoon, and evening, and continue as long as you have any respiratory congestion.

2. When your symptoms are gone, reduce to 6000 mg (5 softgels) twice daily, morning and evening, and continue for three days.

3. At this point you may discontinue Lecithin or continue to take 4800 mg (4 softgels) twice daily, morning and evening, as a maintenance dose to help keep your respiratory system free of congestion.

Remedy At A Glance (Lecithin)

	Morning	Afternoon	Evening
Daily To Relieve Congestion:	6000 mg	6000 mg	6000 mg
Daily For Three Days After You Are Better:	6000 mg		6000 mg
Daily As A Maintenance Dose: (Optional)	4800 mg		4800 mg

See Chapter 9 for more on Lecithin and how to use it to help heal arthritis, prevent bloodclot stroke, lower cholesterol, clean out blocked arteries and heart valves without surgery, prevent arteriosclerosis, end gout, and dissolve gallstones.

Vitamin B12: Use in 1000 mcg tablets, capsules, or sublingual form. Take it with eight ounces of juice or other liquids as directed. (Sublingual form is dissolved under the tongue and requires no liquids.)

1. Take 2000 mcg twice daily, morning and afternoon, and continue until your flu symptoms are gone.

2. Reduce to 1000 mcg twice daily, morning and afternoon, and continue for three days.

3. At this point you may discontinue B12 or continue to take 1000 mcg twice daily, morning and afternoon, as a maintenance dose to help prevent fatigue.

4. Be aware that if you are on bed rest while you have the flu, Vitamin B12 might give you more energy than you want and prevent you from sleeping.

Remedy At A Glance (Vitamin B12)

	Morning	Afternoon
Daily To Relieve Fatigue:	2000 mcg	2000 mcg
Daily For Three Days After You Are Better:	1000 mcg	1000 mcg
Daily As A Maintenance Dose: (Optional)	1000 mcg	1000 mcg

See Chapter 11 for more on Vitamin B12 and how to use it as a remedy to help prevent fatigue and stop tingling extremities.

*   *   *

The following is a case study written as a short story about one of the countless people who have been helped by this remedy: A pharmacist rescues her Aspen honeymoon by using L-Lysine to stop a herpes outbreak just days before her wedding.

"Sleepless"

EIGHT DAYS BEFORE THE WEDDING

Margarite opened her eyes to the darkness and pushed herself to a sitting position, being careful not to move anything below her waist. She leaned back against the small hill of pillows and fished around on top of the end table until she found her lighter, placing the flame next to the wicks of four candles. She watched the candlelight flicker and grow until it cast its amber warmth against the white walls of her bedroom, dancing off the silver bells on the pine wreath hung there. She extracted a cigarette from a pack in the top drawer and noted the time by the lighted green numbers on the clock radio. 4:15 a.m. She'd slept two hours. Even without the aggravation of a herpes outbreak just two days before Christmas, she could never sleep more than four hours at a time. It had been years since she'd slept through the night.

Margarite inhaled deeply twice in succession before placing the cigarette in a glass ashtray. She found the remote tucked between quilt and top sheet and clicked on the television, leaving the sound muted. CNN was airing year-in-review footage of the two state funerals held in September 1997, one in London, the other in Calcutta. She didn't ordinarily hook into mass sentiment, being something of a cynic, but the loss of both these women in the same short period unsettled her in a way she couldn't explain. She watched the split-screen processions as long as she could. Her bladder was full, and she couldn't hold it any longer. She eyed the distance from her brass bed to the bedroom door, and calculated from there to the small blue-tiled bathroom across and down the hall. Not more than fifteen feet. She could make it if she crawled on hands and knees. It would be painful, but not as much as if she tried walking.

This was her worst outbreak in seven years, and she had no idea how she'd first contracted herpes: maybe unprotected sex, or perhaps the latent effect of a childhood disease--neither she nor her twin brother had missed one. She knew she *was* partially to blame for letting it get so bad. She managed the largest twenty-four hour pharmacy in the Hartford area, supervising nine pharmacists and interns, and loved her job because it was the perfect mixture of numbers and chemistry; she was also a Certified Public Accountant. Margarite hesitated to take prescription drugs for herpes because of side effects and the high cost. Unfortunately, over-the-counter remedies didn't help.

She stubbed out the cigarette and threw back the covers. During the twenty minutes it took to crawl to the toilet--stopping repeatedly to rest the insides of her blistered thighs and rear end--relieve herself, and crawl back to bed, she thought about her wedding and tried hard to ignore the pain. She would get her prescription refilled first thing in the morning. Side effects or not, she couldn't function like this. And she had to function. This was her second marriage, and there seemed to be more anticipation, certainly more stress, this time. As she grabbed the brass end post to hoist herself up to the bed, flexing nicely-toned deltoids and biceps, an image flashed before her: she was crawling down the aisle in her cherished white, silk wedding dress, submerged under her lace veil with only the top of her head showing, like an albino turtle.

SIX DAYS BEFORE THE WEDDING

She opened the bathroom door to find Carl waiting just outside. He tried to conceal his concern with a lopsided grin. "My mother's cooking that bad?" he asked. He was a handsome man, tall, with skin the color of Caribbean sand and short brown hair. He was carrying too much weight, but Margarite believed that just made him more loveable, though she was a taut size eight.

She shook her head and forced a small laugh, her auburn eyes opaqued by discomfort. "It's the prescription," she said, resting her shoulder against the door jam. "But it's never made me this sick before." She made a ponytail of her brown hair, using one hand to hold it in place away from her neck, while using the other hand to take a drag on the half-smoked cigarette Carl offered.

"Never have a problem when I use it," Carl said, and leaned forward to kiss her lightly on the mouth.

She pulled away from the kiss and exhaled. "You may want to think twice before you do that. I was on my knees in there," she said, and gestured with her thumb toward the toilet.

"I don't care," he said, and kissed her again. "Yum."

Something in his warm brown eyes and gentle features touched her as it always did, deep inside. She smiled and went into his open arms, wrapping her arms tightly around his neck, feeling the protective security of his love as he surrounded her in his large embrace.

Margarite had started taking her prescription yesterday morning and by evening the blisters no longer hurt. But the fifty dollars she spent for it had been earmarked for her "something blue" garter. And she awoke that morning, Christmas day, to dry heaves and the worst headache of her life. She'd tamed the headache with three Excedrin, but her stomach was still in turmoil.

60

"Do you want to leave?" Carl whispered in her ear.

"No, not at all. I don't want to take you away from your family so early. Your mother went to so much trouble. But I won't be able to eat anything else."

Carl let go of her and said, "Look on the bright side. The herpes is gone, now you won't have to pretend to like Aunt Polly's mincemeat pie."

"What you two doin' up there?" Carl senior called from the bottom of the staircase. "The wedding isn't for another six days. Keep it clean now. Junior, your mother's trying to make me eat Polly's mincemeat. Tastes like week old beef stew."

"I hate it when he calls me that," Carl said. Then in a raised voice, "Okay, Pop. Coming right down."

"But that's all your father ever calls you," Margarite reminded him.

* * *

It started to snow on the drive back to Margarite's place. The truck interior was filled with the tangy smell of roasted turkey, giblet gravy, and bread stuffing, wafting from the shopping bags sent home with them despite their protests. It was more than they could eat in the four days before they left for Aspen. They would have one night alone there before relatives and friends began arriving for the New Year's Eve wedding. Margarite's family and most of her support network were in San Francisco. Only her parents and her brother and his companion would be flying out. She felt a pang in the center of her chest thinking of all the people she wanted to be there who couldn't.

"Thinking about your friends not coming to the wedding?" Carl asked, increasing the wiper speed to compete with snow piling on the windshield.

Margarite moved closer to him on the bench seat but didn't answer. At that moment she was too ashamed to admit she was thinking of one friend in particular. She reached inside the pocket of her down parka to touch the note she still hadn't read. She'd been walking around with it for a week, never finding the right moment to tell Carl. Now is a good time, she reminded herself, but the words stayed in her throat.

Margarite had left work early last Thursday for her final fitting. She was so rushed she didn't notice the note on the windshield until she

61

was in the flow of traffic. Curiosity got the better of her, and she pulled to the shoulder to retrieve it from the passenger-side wiper. When she recognized the signature--the tall angry T hovering over three uncertain letters as though giving them shelter--she started shaking and refolded it without seeing anything but his name. *Thor.* She was overwhelmed by the quantity of emotion she felt and unable to sort out the conflicting nature of her response. All the while amazed that there was any feeling left at all, let alone *so* much. And curious how so much passion could have remained hidden. Surely, it could only be contained by a vessel much larger than she.

"What's the matter," Carl asked, pulling the truck into the driveway and interrupting her thoughts. "Something's been bothering you for a couple of days." He squeezed her hand. "What is it?"

Margarite pretended not to hear, and Carl didn't ask again. He knew she would tell him in her own time, if at all. She knew that had to be soon, that she had to sort out what she still felt for Thor before she married Carl in six days.

She'd only known Thor six days before she'd moved in with him. She had never been happier than she was the first year they'd lived together. She would rush home from work every evening, driving like her life depended on her getting there ten minutes ago, to surge up the steps to the front porch and into his arms.

Thor had mined her heart to a deeper depth of pleasure and her soul to a new level of suffering.

FOUR DAYS BEFORE THE WEDDING

1:30 a.m. Margarite lighted two candles then placed the match's flame at the tip of her cigarette. She was definitely going to cut back after the wedding, she thought, as she inhaled and shook the life from the match. She reached between the mattress and box spring to extract Thor's still-unread note, holding it in her closed fist as she smoked the cigarette. She started to cry suddenly, remembering the last time she'd seen him at Muir Beach.

When the phone rang five years ago she was in the middle of a backyard barbecue, moved indoors because of inclement weather. Her friends were trying to help her forget the trouble that had crept into her seemingly-perfect relationship with Thor. She picked up the receiver, listened for a minute before saying, "okay," then hung up, grabbed her handbag and left without speaking to anyone. She forgot there were people in her house before she shut the door. No explanation was needed. A few sympathetic and knowing glances around the room told the whole story. Thor had said, in the soft clipped voice he used when he wanted something from her, that he could explain everything if she would just come to him. And so she went.

Muir Beach is a fair sized strip of sand separating Muir Woods and Golden Gate National Recreation Area. It took Margarite an hour to get there and another half hour to find the spot he'd indicated on the phone. Thor was waiting at a bench just off one of the nature trails, just inside the woods proper. With his long storybook-blond hair, ocher turtleneck and brown pants, he appeared as one with the new autumn foliage. She almost missed him and turned onto the wrong trail.

"You're late," he growled, as soon as she appeared on the path.

It had rained all morning and the ground was wet and slick. Clumps of mist hung affectionately near the roots of rain-blackened trees.

"Thor, why did we have to meet way out here? Tell you the truth I'd rather be talking over a cappuccino at Starbucks."

When he didn't answer, Margarite approached the bench cautiously and sat down beside him. She knew she shouldn't have come, knew he was already lost to her, knew the trip was mere folly. But she couldn't stop herself. As long as there was any chance of seeing him, even in this newly distorted state, she would take it.

"Are you finished complaining about your little problems, Margo? How many times do I have to tell you? I chose this spot and the other two places, because it's impossible to tape our conversations. The trees, electrical wires, no aluminum alloys, relative dampness of the ground. Unless *you're* wired, that is," he said, and eyed her.

"Thor, for God's sake don't start that again. You really scare me with that kind of talk."

"You're in denial Margo," he said, running his hand across and down her back. "I told you I'm being followed, but you don't want to believe it. That's why I had to move out of the house. The closets were all bugged. I showed you, don't you remember? That's a perfect place to put a bug when you think about it, because no one would ever expect a closet to be bugged."

Margarite said, "How often did we have conversations in the closets?"

His attitude shifted and she tensed.

"People are trying to kill me, poison my food, run me off cliffs, shooting at me--you name it. Got me fired from my last three jobs, one after the other. My life's being ruined."

"By who Thor? You never explain who it is or why they want to hurt *you*."

He stood up and looked around quickly. "They're back, Margo," he said in a hushed tone. "I gotta' go. I'll try to contact you again if they don't kill me first."

"Who's after you, Thor? Who?"

He didn't answer. He simply turned his back and sprinted down the slope to the right of the path, disappearing into the low hanging branches of a stand of evergreens. Margarite watched him run out of her life, chased and dogged by shadows she couldn't perceive. She felt part of her heart cry out at that moment before it shut down in grief.

It didn't help now knowing Thor was again nearby. She returned the note to the mattress and wiped her tears, noting a tingling on the insides of her thighs that meant she was about to have another herpes outbreak.

TWO DAYS BEFORE THE WEDDING

The postman had just made his drop as Margarite returned from her morning run. A good one, four miles. The H-brace she wore on her right leg when running looked odd, but it meant she wouldn't reinjure the knee she'd torn skiing last winter.

"Happy Holidays," the carrier called out as he crossed the driveway pushing a three-wheeled, blue canvas pouch.

"Happy Hanukkah, Mr. Cohen," she said, and he smiled and nodded, appreciating a good Catholic girl who knew the difference.

There were several late Christmas cards in the mail, and she opened them while she ate a bowl of Cheerios laced with three tablespoons of sugar and skim milk. One card was from her auto insurance agent thanking her for her business. One was from Uncle Beau, her mother's brother who still lived in the family homestead in Manchester, England. One had a San Diego postmark, and she smiled when she recognized her good friend's handwriting.

Pictured on the front of the rectangular card were three small African-American angels wearing white choir girl surplices over black cassocks. The third angel, adorned with little auburn Rasta curls, had an impish look on her face--suggesting she had done something she shouldn't--and her halo had drifted askew down the side of her head, confirming the worst. Margarite laughed out loud when she saw it, almost spitting Cheerios across the counter. "Ohmigod, looks exactly like her," she sputtered, and laughed again. She read the handwritten message inside and sat the card in front of her, watching it while she ate, chuckling softly to herself. She poured another bowl of cereal and made a mental note to call Lynn before they left for Aspen that evening, if there was time.

Margarite thought about the book her friend was writing on vitamin remedies, suddenly remembering what she'd told her--*that L-Lysine could stop herpes cold.* As a pharmacist, Margarite had believed the amino acid might prevent a herpes outbreak if taken in advance. What she had not believed was that it was capable of shutting down a full blown case like she currently had. On the other hand, she thought as she burped and tasted sugar, she was ready to try just about anything. She rinsed her bowl and spoon and set them in the sink.

Using a chair to stand on, Margarite reached the top shelf in the pantry and searched the labels for L-Lysine, finding a large bottle bought on Lynn's advice but never opened. She set the bottle on the counter, stepped down, and poured a glass of pink lemonade. Unable to remember how much she was supposed to take, she shrugged, *hell, its only an amino acid,* and poured a handful, swallowing them individually with a big gulp of liquid. When she packed the bottle she noticed the price for 250 was a fraction of what her prescription had cost. The blisters felt better within two hours after taking the first handful of L-Lysine, but she took two more handfuls that day before leaving for the airport.

Thor's note was still tucked ominously inside the left pocket of her parka. Still unread. Each day Margarite imagined that the note became heavier to carry, and she attempted to compensate for this sad burden by carrying a fist-sized rock in the other pocket, one hand grasping the note, the other holding tight to the rock. Why she carried the note without reading it, she didn't know. She was locked in a moment when unproved suspicion threatens to become unwanted discovery. She couldn't destroy the note until she read it, but she couldn't read it. She wasn't strong enough to go forward, out of the safe zone and into the knowing. No matter what the note said, it would mean emotional chaos.

NEW YEAR'S EVE

Margarite studied the full length of her reflection in the antique cheval mirror, pleased with what she saw. From the narrow pointed sleeves to the gold trimmed hem and five foot train, the wedding dress was everything she'd hoped for. No one would ever guess she'd bought it second-hand, she thought and smiled broadly, showing small perfect teeth in a face pinked by a winter tan. Her wholesome skin shone with anticipation and the worry was gone from her eyes, now intoxicated with happiness. She had worked hard to get to this have-it-all moment. Love, health, career. Even the herpes was in remission thanks to the L-Lysine. All she wanted was there for the taking.

She was standing in a small room just off the vestibule at the Chapel of the Angels. Scented trails of rose incense burning in the vestibule snuck under the door. Outside, a Colorado blizzard continued to rage against the walls and windows as dusk closed in. She and Carl had spent most of yesterday digging out members of his family who got stuck driving up the mountain. Everyone took the bad weather with good humor. The worse things became the funnier they seemed and the more they laughed. The forty guests were now seated in the small wood chapel that was decorated with fresh pine boughs, white ribbon bows, hundreds of lighted white candles, and garlands of white flowers.

A knock sounded at the door and her father, Tom, opened it and stuck his head in. "It's time, Margarite," he said, and smiled, coming fully into the room. She walked over and hugged him, the long silk train swishing behind her as she went.

Her mother, Eve, stepped into the room behind Tom. "You look quite beautiful, Margarite Mary," she said, with pride faltering her voice. "But we'd better hurry. Carl is already at the altar. He looks quite handsome in his tuxedo, doesn't he, Tom?"

Tom shrugged. *No man was good enough for his only daughter.*

Margarite said, "You go ahead. I have something to take care of. I'll be out in a minute."

66

She shut the door behind her parents and took her handbag from a hook on the wall. She had moved Thor's note from her parka to her handbag when she changed clothes. Now it was wedged at the bottom of her sunglass case. She pried it out and replaced her handbag on the hook. Margarite held the note, thinking of the two years she'd spent struggling to get over Thor after he disappeared. Remembering how black-hole empty life was until she'd met Carl. Sweet Carl. Without reading it she tore the note in half, again and again. Tore the bigger pieces into smaller pieces and dropped them in a grey plastic waste basket in the corner.

In the petal scented vestibule she took her father's arm and kissed her mother, who left to take her seat, while Margarite and her father took their places at the head of the aisle. As the wedding march began, he turned to her and said, "Life is most often about new beginnings, Margarite. Let go of the past, and it will let go of you."

She smiled, saying, "I think I just figured that out, Daddy." Then she kissed his cheek, and they started down the aisle as the music rose around them.

CHAPTER 5

BETA CAROTENE

•Shorten Healing Time By More Than Half, And _Drastically_ Reduce Wound Tenderness And Scarring

Accelerating The Healing Of *Any Serious Injury*
Preparing For And Quickly Recovering From Surgery
Helping Heal And Prevent Chronic Disorders Like Arthritis And Cancer
Quickly Healing A Temporary Infection Or Inflammation
Preventing And Healing Breast Fibroids
Quickly Healing Cuts, Scrapes, And Minor Injuries

Beta Carotene is one of a group of supplements known as antioxidants that protect cells from free radical damage.[8] Beta Carotene is also the single most important supplement for accelerating all kinds of physical healing. Taken in appropriate dosages, it has miraculous healing powers that have to be witnessed to be believed. For example, if an injury is expected to take two months to heal, Beta Carotene can cut that to four weeks or less. No matter what kind of damage the body sustains, whether it be an accidental injury or recovery

---

8 Free radicals are highly destructive molecules, created when oxygen breaks down and combines with other potentially harmful substances in the body, that can cause extensive damage--from cancer to DNA deviations.

from surgery, Beta Carotene speeds the healing process at an astonishing rate. No matter where the body has been damaged, Beta Carotene can heal in a fraction of the time it would ordinarily take. And it works equally well fighting infection and inflammation.

Beta Carotene also *drastically* reduces wound tenderness and can eliminate most of the redness, swelling, and itching that accompany it. If appropriate levels are taken throughout the healing process, major wounds can result in practically invisible scars.

Recommended Strength[9]

25,000 International Units (IU) (This amount is equal to 15 mg.)

Recommended Form

Softgels *only*

Taken How

As a single dose once a day with your largest meal as directed, regardless of the amount you are taking.

Side Effects

When taking high doses of Beta Carotene, a small number of people experience mild nagging headaches or rashes. These symptoms usually occur only in the first few weeks after beginning the remedy, and end immediately when the remedy is interrupted for a day, or the dosage is lowered. You will know if you have decreased the dosage too much because any injury, infection, or inflammation can worsen within twenty-four hours.

---

9 For Beta Carotene, the author has had the best results with Puritan's Pride®, Oakdale, NY 11769, (800) 645-1030; and Solgar®, Leonia, NJ 07605, (800) 645-2246. Puritan's Pride is available by mail order only. Solgar can be purchased at most health foods stores and sometimes in the health foods section of supermarkets.

√ Beta Carotene can make an injury or wound appear to be healed before it really is. For that reason, it is recommended that you complete all steps of the remedy even if you are feeling no discomfort.

√ When healing a wound, it is not recommended that you apply anything directly to the surface unless your physician has instructed you to. Simply clean the wound once a day with warm water and a mild soap. Keep it dry and covered at all other times.

√ Be alert for a Vitamin D deficiency, which may occur after taking high doses of Beta Carotene for a prolonged period. (Beta Carotene utilizes Vitamin D as it is converted to Vitamin A for the body's use.) The first signs of a Vitamin D deficiency are usually small sores and abrasions on the gums and soft tissue of the mouth. If this happens, stop taking Beta Carotene or lower your dosage for one to two days. Vitamin D can be toxic, and since it generally takes such small amounts to prevent a deficiency, it is not recommended that you use it daily. Keep in mind that most people use Beta Carotene without experiencing a deficiency.

•Shorten Healing Time By More Than Half, And _Drastically_ Reduce Wound Tenderness And Scarring

Accelerating The Healing Of _Any Serious Injury_

1. Take 250,000 IU (10 softgels) of Beta Carotene as soon as possible after the injury, and continue daily for one week.

2. Reduce to 225,000 IU (9 softgels) daily, and continue for two days.

3. Reduce to 200,000 IU (8 softgels) daily, and continue for

five days.

4. Two weeks have passed. Reduce to 175,000 IU (7 softgels) daily, and continue for one week.

5. Reduce to 150,000 IU (6 softgels) daily, and continue for one week.

6. Reduce to 100,000 IU (4 softgels) daily, and continue for two weeks.

7. Six weeks have passed. At this point you may discontinue Beta Carotene or continue to take 50,000 IU (2 softgels) daily, as a maintenance dose to help maintain optimum health in bone and soft tissue.

Remedy At A Glance (Beta Carotene)

	Once A Day With Largest Meal	
Daily First Week To Relieve Symptoms:	250,000 IU	
	Days 1-2	Days 3-7
Daily Second Week To Relieve Symptoms:	225,000 IU	200,000 IU
Daily Third Week To Relieve Symptoms	175,000 IU	
Daily Fourth Week To Relieve Symptoms:	150,000 IU	
Daily Fifth And Sixth Weeks To Relieve Symptoms:	100,000 IU	
Daily As A Maintenance Dose: (Optional)	50,000 IU	

Notes√√

√ Beta Carotene works best when taken with food; ordinarily, it should be taken as a single dose with your largest meal. If you are not

72

eating regular meals because of a serious injury, take it with eight ounces of juice or other liquids. If possible, avoid taking it with water.

√ Remember, if your injury starts to bother you again--pain, tenderness, swelling, itching, redness, or any other discomfort--after you have reduced your daily dosage, increase it back up to the level that brought you relief.

Preparing For And Quickly Recovering From Surgery

1. Beginning two days before surgery and continuing five days after, take 250,000 IU of Beta Carotene daily. On the day of surgery, take it as soon as possible after the procedure.

2. Follow steps 2-7 above for, "Speeding The Healing Of *Any Serious Injury*."

Remedy At A Glance (Beta Carotene)

Once A Day With Largest Meal

Beginning Two Days Before Surgery And Continuing Five Days After

	Days 1-2	Days 3-7
Daily The Week Of Surgery:	250,000 IU	
Daily Second Week To Relieve Symptoms:	225,000 IU	200,000 IU
Daily Third Week To Relieve Symptoms	175,000 IU	
Daily Fourth Week To Relieve Symptoms:	150,000 IU	
Daily Fifth And Sixth Weeks To Relieve Symptoms:	100,000 IU	
Daily As A Maintenance Dose: (Optional)	50,000 IU	

Helping Heal And Prevent Chronic Disorders Like Arthritis And Cancer--Other disorders that can also benefit from this remedy are: allergies, angina, arteriosclerosis, asthma, bladder infection, breast fibroids, bronchitis, bursitis, Crohn's disease, hemorrhoids, infection and inflammation, inflammatory bowel disease, intestinal disorders, nagging cough, repetitive stress disorders, respiratory illnesses, sinus problems, stroke, tendonitis, etc.

1. Take 250,000 IU (10 softgels) of Beta Carotene daily for the first two days of each week, i.e. Sunday and Monday.

2. Reduce to 200,000 IU (8 softgels) daily for the next three days, i.e., Tuesday, Wednesday, and Thursday.

3. Reduce to 150,000 IU (6 softgels) daily for the last two days, i.e., Friday and Saturday.

4. Continue this weekly schedule until your symptoms are gone, then reduce to 100,000 IU (4 softgels) daily, and continue as a maintenance dose whether or not you are experiencing symptoms.

Remedy At A Glance (Beta Carotene)

	Days 1-2	Days 3-5	Days 6-7
Daily To Relieve Symptoms:	250,000 IU	200,000 IU	150,000 IU
Daily As A Maintenance Dose:	100,000 IU		

Notes√√

√ To help heal and prevent colon cancer, Crohn's disease, inflammatory bowel disease, or any other intestinal disorder, it is recommended that you also take **Acidophilus** and edible **Aloe Vera Gel**. Both help to promote good health throughout the entire intestinal tract.

Acidophilus: Use a formula that contains active lactobacillus, measured in the millions. Use in softgel or capsule form. Take it a half hour before you eat, with eight ounces of juice or other liquids as directed.

1. Take one softgel or capsule every other day in the morning, and continue as a maintenance dose to promote good health in your intestinal tract.

2. To avoid creating an imbalance, stop taking Acidophilus for one week each month.

Remedy At A Glance (Acidophilus)

Every Other Day As A Maintenance Dose (Three Out Of Four Weeks Only):	Morning
	One Capsule Or Softgel

See Chapter 8 for more on Acidophilus and how to use it as a remedy to heal vaginal itching, yeast infection, and toenail fungus.

Edible Aloe Vera Gel: Use in liquid form.[10] Take it on an empty stomach, followed by eight ounces of water.

1. Take one tablespoon daily, and continue as a maintenance dose to promote good health in your intestinal tract.

---

10 The author has had the best results with Puritan's Pride® edible Aloe Vera Gel, Oakdale, NY 11769, available by mail order only at (800) 645-1030.

75

Remedy At A Glance (Edible Aloe Vera Gel)

√ To help heal asthma, chronic bronchitis, nagging cough, or other respiratory disorders, it is recommended that you also take **L-Cysteine** and **Vitamin C Complex**. This combination can work wonders in promoting good health in lung tissue. If you have congestion, you should also take **Lecithin**.

L-Cysteine And Vitamin C Complex Taken Together In Combination: Use 500 mg tablets or capsules of L-Cysteine; use 1000 mg tablets or capsules of Vitamin C Complex. They should be taken together--at the same time--with juice or other liquids as directed. The amount of Vitamin C Complex should always equal twice that of L-Cysteine.

1. Take 1000 mg of L-Cysteine and 2000 mg of Vitamin C Complex (a "double dose") four times daily, i.e., 8:00 am, noon, 4:00 pm, 8:00 pm, and continue until your symptoms are gone.

2. Reduce to a double dose three times daily, morning, afternoon, and evening, and continue for four weeks.

3. Continue to take a double dose twice daily, morning and evening, as a maintenance dose to help maintain good health in your respiratory system.

Remedy At A Glance (L-Cysteine And Vitamin C Complex)

	8:00 am	Noon	4:00 pm	8:00 pm
Daily To Relieve Symptoms:	Double Dose	Double Dose	Double Dose	Double Dose
	Morning	Afternoon	Evening	
Daily For Four Weeks After You Are Better:	Double Dose	Double Dose	Double Dose	
Daily As A Maintenance Dose :	Double Dose		Double Dose	

See Chapter 3 for more on L-Cysteine and Vitamin C Complex and how to use this powerful combination to guard against cigarette smoker's damage, to prevent hangovers, to avoid liver/age spots, and to protect against environmental toxins.

Lecithin: Use in 1200 mg softgels only. Take it with eight ounces of juice or other liquids as directed. (Chapter 9 tells you how to use the granular form to supplement your daily doses.)

1. Take 6000 mg (5 softgels) three times daily, morning, afternoon, and evening, and continue as long as you have congestion.

2. Reduce to 6000 mg (5 softgels) twice daily, morning and evening, and continue for four weeks.

3. Continue to take 4800 mg (4 softgels) twice daily, as a maintenance dose to help prevent congestion.

Remedy At A Glance (Lecithin)

	Morning	Afternoon	Evening
Daily To Clear Up Congestion:	6000 mg	6000 mg	6000 mg
Daily For Four Weeks After You Are Better:	6000 mg		6000 mg
Daily As A Maintenance Dose:	4800 mg		4800 mg

See Chapter 9 for more on Lecithin and how to use it to help heal arthritis, prevent bloodclot stroke, lower cholesterol, clean out blocked arteries and heart valves without surgery, prevent arteriosclerosis, end gout, and dissolve gallstones.

√ If you have arthritis, please see Chapter 9, for how to help heal and lessen the effects of this disorder with additional supplements. There is too much information to include as a note here.

Quickly Healing A Temporary Infection Or Inflammation

1. Take 250,000 IU (10 softgels) of Beta Carotene daily, beginning on the first day of your ailment, and continue for up to five days.

2. If you still have symptoms after the fifth day, reduce to 200,000 IU (8 softgels) daily, and continue at this level until your symptoms are gone.

3. Reduce to 100,000 (4 softgels) daily, and continue for three days.

4. At this point you may discontinue Beta Carotene or continue to take 50,000 IU (2 softgels) daily, as a maintenance dose to help promote good health in bone and soft tissue.

Remedy At A Glance (Beta Carotene)

	Once A Day With Largest Meal
Daily For First Five Days To Relieve Symptoms:	250,000 IU
Daily After Fifth Day To Relieve Symptoms:	200,000 IU
Daily For Three Days After You Are Better:	100,000 IU
Daily As A Maintenance Dose: (Optional)	50,000 IU

See Chapter 4 for more on L-Lysine and how to use it to help heal herpes, cold sores, flu, and other viruses.

See Chapter 7 for more on Bee Pollen and Vitamin C Complex and how to use the combination to help heal colds, allergies, and sinus problems.

See Chapter 8 for more on Acidophilus and how to use it to help heal yeast infection, vaginal itching, and toenail fungus.

Quickly Healing Cuts, Scrapes, And Minor Injuries

1. Take 250,000 IU (10 softgels) of Beta Carotene directly after the injury, and again on the following day.

2. Reduce to 200,000 IU (8 softgels) daily, and continue until your symptoms are gone.

3. Reduce to 100,000 IU (4 softgels) daily, and continue for three days.

4. At this point you may discontinue Beta Carotene, or continue to take 50,000 IU (2 softgels) daily, as a maintenance dose to maintain optimum health in bone and soft tissue.

Remedy At A Glance (Beta Carotene)

	Once A Day With Largest Meal
Daily First Two Days To Relieve Symptoms:	250,000 IU
Daily To Relieve Symptoms:	200,000 IU
Daily For Three Days After You Are Better:	100,000 IU
Daily As A Maintenance Dose: (Optional)	50,000 IU

*   *   *

The following is a case study written as a short story about one of the countless people who have been helped by this remedy: A Manhattan journalist uses Beta Carotene to speed heal a stab wound when celebrity worship of a Stallone look-alike erupts in violence.

"Only A Picture Image"

Ron edged his face closer to Kim's in the confined space of the car. They were in the front seat of his brown station wagon in the pre-dawn hours of a muggy August morning. She ignored the little voice of instinct coaxing her to open the door and run away. She sat as though charmed as Ron pulled a serrated steak knife out of the glove compartment, still wrapped in cellophane, with an orange price tag stuck to the handle. She noted absently that it sold for $4.99.

Kim stared into Ron's face. It was the face she loved, the one she saw in her dreams, in the movies too. She'd watched him strut across the stage to win a Sylvester Stallone look-alike contest in Asbury Park just that summer; wrote a human interest piece on it for her paper. Ron's face was broader than Mr. Stallone's, but otherwise the two men shared the same features and mannerisms--though Ron's words didn't spill out of the side of his mouth. And there were other small differences.

Stallone was the first man Kim wanted when she ripened. She began creating sexual fantasies about the star the summer her parents divorced. She was fourteen. She and her cousin Heather saw *Lords Of Flatbush* right before relocating to the summer home at White Rock Lake. Every afternoon the girls snuck off to a small wooded area to sit with their narrow backs leaning against the trunk of a large evergreen. The floor of dead brown needles muffled their young laughter, while they shared cigarettes stolen from Endira, the Mexican cook. They held the cigarettes like specimens between thumb and index finger, inhaling shallow draws, exciting themselves with lewd talk about the actor. As an adult, Kim secretly compared all other men to him.

Then one rainy Friday night last November, the day after Thanksgiving, Ron had walked into Ida's Bar where Kim was drinking with friends after work. She had volunteered to pick up the check, as usual, and was sipping her third Johnny Walker Black on ice. The jukebox was playing Olivia Newton-John's serene, "Hopelessly Devoted To You." Across the room, a Puerto Rican couple danced in a slow circle next to their table. Kim lit a cigarette and gazed through the hazy smoke toward the front.

And there he was.

Standing very still.

He confidently surveyed the room, one hand in the pocket of his chinos, the other holding an unlighted cigarette. Tiny rain drops shimmered on top of his thick, dark hair and across the shoulders of his leather bomber's jacket. Kim was reminded of Johnny Kovak in *F.I.S.T.*, casing a new neighborhood before settling down to recruit for his trucker's union.

Ron's eyes found Kim's and held them tenderly. He smiled and nodded, accepting the unspoken invitation before turning to find a spot at the bar.

Kim's mind reeled as she fumbled with her gold lighter, touching the flame to the already-glowing tip of her cigarette. She had removed her contact lenses after work, and with the help of the scotch, believed that Stallone had actually walked into the bar. This *was* New York City; they *were* only thirty blocks or so from The Carlyle where he sometimes stayed.

Alkai, a bookkeeper at Hearst Publishing where they both worked, saw the look of utter stupefaction in Kim's hazel eyes and turned her large body to find its source. She understood immediately. Ron's face was visible in the gold-specked mirror lining the wall behind the liquor bottles, and he was watching them. She turned back to Kim.

"Oh gawd. I hope you know that's not really Sylvester Stallone standing ova' there at the bar," she said. "Just lookit' that gut, and he's too tall. Not to mention Stallone wouldn't be found dead here." Her speech was a mixture of the Philippines and east Bronx.

Rwanda, the sixty-something receptionist with cola-colored skin, saw the disappointment on Kim's features and added, "Maybe he's a relative. D'ya wanna send him a drink?"

The jukebox fell silent for a moment before Tina Turner's luscious voice began singing, "*May seem to you that I'm acting confused when you're close to me.*" Kim slipped her red-framed glasses out of her handbag, put them on, and glanced hopefully toward the bar. "*Whatever the rea-son, you do it for me.*" She decided, as she put away her glasses, that Ron was close enough to the real thing, and that she would take Rwanda's suggestion about the drink. "*What's love got to do, got to do with it?*"

Two hours later, Ron went home with Kim and stayed until Sunday afternoon. It rained hard all weekend, but that wasn't why they had stayed in. Since then, they met every Friday at Ida's and spent three out of four weekends at Kim's Tudor City apartment. In that time she had learned little more than Ron Richard's name. She had no way of contacting him except at Ida's, on Friday's. And Kim didn't care. At least not at the start. She didn't know that exploring Ron's world would shrink and distort her own.

The argument that began earlier inside Ida's had been over nothing, really. It was even a bit romantic--their first quarrel. They'd been drinking for hours, with Kim asking the usual questions, when words turned to shouts. When her frustration peaked, she poured her drink over Ron's head and watched it run down in tiny rivulets, staining his white shirt and grey blazer. But that wasn't what closed his face. It was what she said after that, but whatever it was she couldn't remember. Matters escalated quickly: Joey, the hefty bartender-bouncer who worked days at the dock with his Uncle Louie, asked them to leave. When they took too long settling up, arguing about who owed what, he and another associate assisted them outside, despite Ron's loud threats to sue and Kim's equally noisy assertions that she'd been thrown out of better places. (True, but Ida's was her favorite bar in New York City.)

Kim had Ron's car keys and she walked off quickly with her sandals flapping lightly against the pavement. Ron stood in front arguing with Joey who didn't say a word, waiting for Ron to start something he couldn't finish.

When Ron caught up with Kim ten minutes later, breathing hard, he discovered she had locked herself inside his car. *She would show him.* Talking through a one inch gap she left at the top of the passenger window, Ron tried to convince her to unlock the door. His words sounded sincere, but his eyes were opaque. Kim refused. After several minutes of pleading Ron lost his composure, lifted his right leg and kicked the passenger window hard. The glass spiderwebbed but didn't shatter. Kim slid over quickly to sit behind the steering wheel with her back pressed against the driver's door, feeling thrilled. Ron continued to kick the window until it collapsed into pieces. He reached in to unlock the door and got in, unmindful of broken glass on the seat.

"What are you doing?" Kim whispered, as Ron tore the cellophane from the knife. A street lamp cast a melancholy light through the windshield that glinted off the five-inch blade. It had a black handle with small grooves for finger grips and belonged in a well-equipped kitchen.

Kim felt as if she were watching from far away.

"You went too far this time, Kim," Ron threatened in a soft voice.

"Why didn't you just tell me you were married?" she cried out, trying to loosen the fear that clung to her back and menaced her shoulders. "Then I wouldn't have had to find out for myself, seen that yard with those damned pink ducks wading through yellow daisies." Her Texas accent was thick with emotion. Then she remembered, That was what she said inside! What told Ron she'd pierced his cover, had tracked him to Long Island, to his wife and three children. The remark sent him into a renewed panic, and he moved the knife closer to Kim.

"What are you doing?" she asked again, unable to think of anything else to say. Terror was constricting her breathing. Her voice sounded thin and breathless to her own ears.

"I'm going to cut you now Kim so you'll remember to never go near my family again," he said evenly, like a teacher instructing a student.

83

Kim was wondering if Ron could hurt her so casually--weren't they in love?--when he leaned in and thrust the knife at her. She jerked her right arm back and to the side, deflecting the force of the attack into her upper arm instead of her rib cage. The knife left a vertical three-inch gash an inch deep. Kim whimpered but didn't cry out, not even when blood began seeping urgently down her arm.

A police car and two fire trucks raced past, their sirens ebbing with distance until a New York silence settled again over the street.

Finally Ron reacted, "Oh God, what have I done?"

He reached into the back seat and grabbed a wad of Kleenex, pressed it against the wound and instructed Kim to hold the tissues in place with her other hand. He took a necktie out of his blazer pocket and tied it around the Kleenex bandage. Then he removed his Armani belt, a birthday present from Kim, and tied it around her upper arm to staunch the flow of blood. Kim still hadn't spoken and wasn't crying. She sat quietly while he performed his ministrations, tasting bile at the top of her throat but saying nothing. Ron finished and looked up into Kim's amber-specked eyes ablaze with anger. Suddenly, he felt a crushing sense of loss and began to cry in wracking sobs. She watched him, thinking, He even cries like Stallone, and recalled John Rambo in the final scene of *First Blood*.

"I'm so sorry. Oh God. I didn't mean to do it. I swear I didn't mean to hurt you like this. But why did you have to go near my family? I can't let you hurt my family." He wiped his eyes with a tissue and blew his nose before asking, "What should we do now?"

Kim studied Ron while blood seeped slowly through the wad of tissues, staining her yellow sundress a sickening red-orange. Her thoughts were softening around the edges, a haze was growing over the moment. It was being wrapped in white tissue paper so she could take it home with her. A chill crawled up Kim's back and she turned away to get out of the car. Ron slid over and followed her out the door, showering bits of glass on the asphalt. It was 4:00 Saturday morning. Kim stared blankly toward Second Avenue where traffic flowed south, headed for the Queens Midtown Tunnel. A warm breeze blowing across 42nd Street rustled the damp hair on the back of her neck.

"Kim. I ... I ... ahh, don't know what to do--I mean ... should I ...? What should I do Kim?"

She watched him, cradling her wounded right arm with her

good one, wondering what Stallone would do here. But Stallone would never be here. Rocky Balboa would never hurt a woman. She felt lightheaded and cold through to the bone, even though the temperature hovered in the high 80s. She sat down shakily on the curb, dropping her head between her knees, surprised that her wounded arm didn't hurt more. Blood was in her shoulder-length blonde hair and under her manicured red nails. It stuck her toes to her white sandals.

Ron came and stood over her, while small helpless gestures played on his hands. He asked again what to do. Kim looked up at him, hunched and uncertain, and felt the full weight of her fantasy.

She said, "You should get in you car and go home, Ron. Go home to your f---ing pink ducks wading through yellow daises."

"Are you sure that'd be okay?" he asked, without irony.

Kim was struck anew but nodded slowly.

Relief softened the lines that had worried Ron's forehead. "Okay then. I'll see you next Friday," he said, and walked to his station wagon crunching broken glass underfoot. He drove off without looking back.

Watching Ron's taillights recede made her feel as if it were she who was getting smaller, not the car. She felt completely alone. How could he not know what to do? Damn Yankee.

After only a moment to feel sorry for herself, Kim stood slowly, cradling her right arm, and walked west toward Second Avenue. She hailed a cab without difficulty, unusual at that time of the morning. The driver began writing on his clipboard as soon as he stopped. He didn't notice Kim's condition until she was inside.

"Come on lady," he pleaded, looking at her in the rear view mirror. "Regulations not permit me to transport sick people. You call 911. Is the law." Passengers on their way to emergency rooms rarely tipped and often left the upholstery sticky. The driver shrugged his bony shoulders and waited. He was Eastern European, in his fifties, and smelled of stale tobacco.

Kim took a deep breath and leaned forward, talking through the open door in the metal grate separating the front seat from the back, offering the driver a modicum of protection from his passengers.

"Listen, you jerk. Take me to New York Medical Center now, 'cause no way am I getting out of this cab. And the quicker you get me there the less blood you'll have to clean up later." She squinted to read the driver's name on the hack license attached to the right side of the dashboard. "There's a twenty-dollar tip in it for you, Igor. That's about two dollars a block. Now move it."

Kim didn't know what she would do next if Igor refused, but the twenty dollars warmed his heart in a way her plight couldn't. He pulled away from the curb with a squeal of rubber, narrowly missing two other cabs cutting into his lane. She was thrown heavily against the seat and choked down a wave of nausea rising in her throat. She laid her head back, breathing through her mouth, and closed her eyes on a burning pain beginning in her arm. At the ER she told police she didn't know the man who attacked her. When they asked her about the silk necktie and Armani belt, she couldn't think of an explanation, and the officers didn't press her.

*   *   *

When I answered the bedside phone at eight that morning, Kim was explaining what was wrong before I could say hello. Her voice was trembling and she sounded close to tears.

"I am such a dumbs---. I cannot believe the way I acted. You warned me not to tell him what we found out," she said. "I asked for it. I really did."

She continued in this manner until I pieced together the story.

When Kim finished I felt bad. Without my help she wouldn't have gotten a look at those pink ducks. It was my idea to track Ron through the DMV using a phony traffic accident, because the plate number and make of his car were all Kim knew other than his name. I drove her out to Hempstead, Long Island, because she was too rattled to drive safely; and because I didn't want her to have to face the knowing alone. Over time she'd become obsessed with finding out about Ron, who had hinted that he was a CIA agent, and the secret brother of Sylvester Stallone. (We learned later that he repaired escalators.)

Kim said she was back at her apartment and wanted my help changing the bandage and cleaning her wound. It had to be done once a day for the next week.

"In a few days I'll be able to do it myself, but I'm a little shaky now," she explained unnecessarily.

I told her I'd be there as soon as I could.

I hung up and tried to scrub off my complicity in a hot shower, then pulled on cut-off jeans, white tee and sneakers. In the kitchen, I spent the next hour chopping fresh vegetables and cubing chicken breasts for soup and teriyaki salad. I also made scratch biscuits. I could at least offer Kim the contentment of a full stomach. I grabbed an unopened bottle of Beta Carotene and put everything in a shopping bag. As soon as I arrived at Kim's, I warmed a bowl of soup on the stove top and served it to her with biscuits. After she ate, I gave her 250,000 International Units of Beta Carotene.

Kim's gash wasn't sewn shut, just taped closed. When she removed the tape to show me, I felt slightly sick and had to sit down. The cut was deep and exposed the separate layers of the epidermis beneath the skin, as it might be seen in a medical textbook. I drove her back to the ER to have the wound cleaned by a professional. I couldn't look at it again.

Later we stopped at a small, private park across the street from Kim's apartment before going upstairs. She unlocked the tall wrought-iron gate and we settled on a bench under a crab apple tree and watched three squirrels scatter for food. They were joined by several sparrows claiming a share. The breeze was spiced with the tart, sugary smell of overripe apples. I parted my lips and tasted the spicy air with my tongue, letting it sting the corners of my jaw.

"I feel like I'm in a Disney movie," Kim said, and we laughed, grateful for the opportunity. The silence stretched as we enjoyed the moment.

Without warning, she reached into her shoulder bag, plucked a hundred-dollar bill from her wallet and put it in my hand.

"What's this for?" I asked.

"To pay for the food and the vitamins. You're a student, you don't have it to spend."

"I won't argue with that, but the cost of what I brought down is about twenty dollars."

"Keep the rest of it to get you through the week," she insisted. "You need it. You'd do the same for me. Besides, look around, who else do you see here cooking for me and taking care of me? Why shouldn't I give it to you?"

"I appreciate this Kim. Really. But are you sure you can afford it?"

"I have extra income from a small trust fund. I can afford it."

"In that case, thank you. You're right, I *can* use it," I said, and folded the crisp new bill before tucking it into my back pocket. "But if you have that kind of money why do you work?"

"I could have five million in the bank and I'd still work every day," she said. "I don't feel right unless I have a job. You never know what could happen."

After pausing she turned her head to look directly at me, "You're wondering why I'm not more upset, aren't you?" she asked, and before I could respond, she explained. "It's because I think I created that scene and got just what I deserved. Has nothing to do with you. It was my decision to act on the information you gave me. I had no business spying on him. He never made me any promises."

"How could you be responsible for a man stabbing you and leaving you alone on 42nd Street at four in the morning? Doesn't Ron bear part of the responsibility? You didn't stab yourself."

"I told him it was okay to leave."

I took a deep breath and counted to ten before saying, "You know, it's possible to assume too much responsibility."

"What do you mean? Besides, what can I do, stab him back?"

"No, but you could swear out a complaint, tell the cops the truth. You know the name of your attacker."

She shook her head. "I love Ron. I don't want anything bad to happen to him."

"He could have killed you, Kim. And don't tell me you provoked him 'cause I don't want to hear it."

The conversation ended then and we went inside. On the ride up to the ninth floor I thought that, despite my carping, I was still impressed by Kim's attitude. She was tough and capable. Upstairs, we ate steaming hot soup with biscuits and salad. While I washed the dishes, she took the phone to the far end of the studio and called the police.

Two hours after she spoke to Detective Silverano, Ron was arrested at his home. When he answered the door and saw the uniforms and flashing lights, he was flooded with relief. He'd never hurt a woman before. He'd intended just to prick Kim's skin, draw a little blood and scare her off his family. At the age of two days he had been left on the steps of St. Anthony's Orphanage. The nuns had tried to give him a good life, but the family in Hempstead was the only one he'd ever had. He was released from Riker's Island five days later, and went home to explain to his wife.

Kim was already taking several vitamins and she easily included Beta Carotene into her daily regimen. Her wound healed remarkably fast, causing her intern to sew it closed sooner than he expected. He actually had to cut the wound open, because part of it had closed early. On two occasions the wound appeared to be healed, and Kim stopped the remedy only to experience a worsening of the injury within two days. It turned red and started to itch and throb, until she returned to the Beta Carotene--which brought relief within the next eight hours. After six weeks on the remedy, Kim's scar had smoothed to a thin line a fraction of the size of the original wound.

While Kim's arm healed and later when she no longer really needed my help, I continued to cook and bring food down to her. Sometimes we'd shop at Greenbergs or Gristedes and cook at her place. She hadn't mentioned Ron, but a soiled work shirt hanging on the back of the bathroom door told me she was seeing him again.

One evening in early December, we were preparing marinara sauce in her tiny kitchen when Kim announced, "I've got a surprise for you my friend. How'd you like to go to Cozumel for two weeks? An island in the Mexican Caribbean? 80 degrees? Sunshine? You remember sunshine, don't you?"

I stopped with my knife poised over the tomatoes. Kim was beaming as she wiped her hands on blue-jeaned thighs and pulled an envelope out of a drawer beneath the counter. Inside were two round-trip tickets and itineraries from Mexicana Airlines.

I grabbed the tickets out of her hand and let out a shriek. I'd never been to Mexico.

CHAPTER 6

COENZYME Q10

•Stop Panic Disorders From Controlling Your Life
Lessening The Severity Of Panic Attack Disorders
Lowering Performance Anxiety
Gaining More Emotional Control In Your Daily Life

•Help Alleviate Long-Term Fatigue And Increase Endurance
Regaining Your Strength And Building A Reserve

Coenzyme Q10 (CoQ10) is an antioxidant which is found throughout the cells and tissues of all oxygen-dependent life forms. Without it the body is incapable of producing energy. In many cases, CoQ10 has the paradoxical ability to greatly increase energy levels without causing mania, while simultaneously decreasing anxiety levels without causing depression. Most people who try CoQ10 report higher energy levels accompanied by a luxurious calm which can lead to a greater degree of emotional control and a significant decrease in panic disorders.

CoQ10 can help calm and balance the adrenal system, which is responsible for the symptoms that signal the onset of a panic disorder: unbridled fear, racing or irregular heartbeat, hot flashes, inability to speak, nausea, vomiting, disorientation, feelings of unreality, tunnel vision, diarrhea, inability to swallow, bright visual spots, heavy sweats, fear of leaving home, etc. If you experience panic not associated with a specific threat, it can be due to an inappropriate adrenal response-- your body preparing to fight or run, when there is no need for either reaction.

For many people, CoQ10 helps suppress the inappropriate

triggering of the fight or flight reaction to nonthreatening circumstances. If you suffer from panic attacks that keep you at home or that occur without warning or reason, CoQ10 can greatly lessen these attacks and in some cases eliminate them. If you experience performance anxiety beyond normal nervousness, CoQ10 can substantially reduce this excessive anxiety. It can also help you gain more emotional control in routine personal situations.

Recommended Strength[11]

30 mg (ubiquinone)

Recommended Form

Capsules only

Taken How

With eight ounces of juice or other liquids as directed.

Side Effects

None observed when taken as directed.

Notes√√

√ CoQ10 usually has to accumulate in the body before its benefits can be perceived. It can take four to six weeks of daily use before the beneficial effects are noticeable.

---

11 The author has had the best results with <u>Country Life®</u>, Coenzyme Q10, Hauppauge, NY 11799, (800) 645-5768, available at most health food stores and sometimes in the health foods section of supermarkets.

•Stop Panic Disorders From Controlling Your Life

Lessening The Severity Of Panic Attack Disorders

Lowering Performance Anxiety

Gaining More Emotional Control In Your Daily Life

1. Take 30 mg of CoQ10 twice daily, morning and afternoon, and continue for five weeks.

2. Reduce to 30 mg once a day in the morning, and continue as a maintenance dose to help prevent your symptoms.

Remedy At A Glance (Coenzyme Q10)

	Morning	Afternoon
Daily For Five Weeks To Relieve Symptoms:	30 mg	30 mg
Daily As A Maintenance Dose:	30 mg	

Notes√√

√ To help prevent and lessen the severity of panic disorders, it is recommended that you also take **Kava Kava**, because it can greatly relieve stress and anxiety.

Kava Kava (Piper Methysticum): Use a root extract formula that contains from thirty to fifty-five percent kavalactones.[12] Look for percentages on the label, because formulas vary among manufacturers: a 250 milligram formula may have a higher percentage of kavalactones than a 300 milligram formula. Use capsules or softgels only. Take it with juice or other liquids as directed.

1. Take two capsules or softgels in the morning, and one in the early afternoon, and continue as a maintenance dose to help lessen anxiety and stress.

2. Extended daily use of Kava Kava can cause dry, flaky skin and itching. For this reason, it is important not to exceed the recommended daily dosages. If you experience these symptoms, add one tablespoon of extra-virgin olive oil to your daily diet, used directly from the bottle--not in cooking. Wait a few days and see if this alleviates your dry skin. If not, you will have to decrease your daily intake of Kava Kava below that recommended here.

Remedy At A Glance (Kava Kava)

	Morning	Afternoon
Daily To Relieve Stress:	2 Softgels or Capsules	1 Softgel or Capsule

See Volume II of this series for more on Kava Kava and how to use it as a remedy to fight stress and anxiety.

---

12 For Kava Kava the author has had the best results with Enzymatic Therapy® ("Kava-55"), Green Bay, WI 54311, (800) 783-2286, (en espanol (800) 552-6338); and Solaray®, Park City, UT 84068. They are available at most health foods stores and sometimes in the health foods section of supermarkets.

•Help Alleviate Long-Term Fatigue And Increase Endurance

Regaining Your Strength And Building A Reserve

1. Take 30 mg of CoQ10 twice daily, morning and afternoon, and continue for four weeks.

2. Reduce to 30 mg once a day in the morning, and continue as a maintenance dose to help maintain increased endurance.

Remedy At A Glance (Coenzyme Q10)

	Morning	Afternoon
Daily For Four Weeks To Relieve Symptoms:	30 mg	30 mg
Daily As A Maintenance Dose:	30 mg	

Notes√√

√ To help relieve fatigue it is recommended that you also take **Vitamin B12**. It increases the flow of oxygen to all parts of your body and can make you feel more energized and alert within hours.

Vitamin B12: Use in 1000 mcg tablets, capsules, or sublingual form. Take it with eight ounces of juice or other liquids as directed. (Sublingual is dissolved under the tongue and requires no liquids.)

1. Take 2000 mcg twice daily, morning and afternoon, and continue for six weeks.

2. Reduce to 2000 mcg in the morning, and 1000 mcg in the afternoon, and continue for two weeks.

3. Continue to take 1000 mcg twice daily, morning and afternoon, as a maintenance dose to help prevent fatigue.

Remedy At A Glance (Vitamin B12)

	Morning	Afternoon
Daily For Six Weeks To Relieve Fatigue:	2000 mcg	2000 mcg
Daily For Two Weeks To Relieve Fatigue:	2000 mcg	1000 mcg
Daily As A Maintenance Dose:	1000 mcg	1000 mcg

See Chapter 11 for more on Vitamin B12 and how to use it as a remedy to help prevent fatigue and stop tingling extremities.

√ If you take Vitamin B12 for more than a few days at a time, it is recommended that you also take **Vitamin B Complex**, to avoid depleting other elements of the B Complex and causing a different deficiency than the one you are treating. You do not have to take B Complex and B12 together--at the same time. Be aware that B Complex can turn urine a darker yellow due to the concentration of nutrients present in B vitamins, and this is not cause for alarm.

Vitamin B Complex: Use B Complex 100, tablets or capsules.[13] (Some B vitamins included in the 100 complex are measured in milligrams, others in micrograms, but all will be contained in one tablet or capsule.) Vitamin B Complex is available in higher strength formulas, up to B Complex 150, and you may use a higher strength formula if you wish. Take it with food, because it can be hard to digest.

---

13 For Vitamin B Complex, the author has had the best results with Country Life®, Hauppauge, NY 11788, (800) 645-5768; Puritan's Pride®, Oakdale, NY 11769, (800) 645-1030; and Solgar®, Leonia, NJ 07605, (800) 645-2246. Puritan's Pride is available by mail order only. The other brands can be purchased at most health foods stores and sometimes in the health foods section of supermarkets.

1. Take one tablet or capsule once a day, and continue as a maintenance dose as long as you take Vitamin B12.

Remedy At A Glance (Vitamin B Complex)

Daily As A Maintenance Dose While Taking B12:	Once A Day With Food
	B Complex 100 or higher

See Volume II of this series for more on Vitamin B Complex and how to use it as a remedy for certain kinds of nervousness, including muscle tics and trembling in your extremities.

*   *   *

The following is a case study written as a short story about one of the countless people who have been helped by this remedy: A first year Ivy League law student uses CoQ10 to help control performance anxiety when facing a professor seeking revenge.

"The Petition"

I am too embarrassed to call 911, thinking how uncool it would be, as I lay slumped against the wall in a corner just inside my apartment next to the door--in fetal position with knees against my chest hugging the phone. Knowing how highly my fellow law students prize cool, I dial Mary's number instead. She picks up on the second ring.

"I think I'm having a heart attack," I say in a hoarse whisper, unable to take in enough air to speak clearly, my chest and neck muscles so tight I think I might suffocate. "But maybe not. Talk to me. Help me calm down." When I finish I am out of breath, sucking air in short little gasps, my body shivering--chilled through with an all abiding fear.

Mary is saying, "What makes you think you're having a heart attack?" and I realize she's been repeating the question.

"Lynn, why do you think you're having a heart attack?"

I search for an answer and realize I don't know.

"Are you having chest pains or pain in either arm?" Mary asks.

"No. But I feel *so* awful," is all I can say, and now I start to cry, because I know I'm going to die.

"We better call 911. Do you want me to do it? Hang up. I'll do it," Mary says, taking control. "I'm coming over after I call. If I miss you, I'll meet you in the ER."

I don't answer right away. Then, "I'm afraid to hang up."

Mary saying, "Lynn, you're going to be all right," talking softly now, the authority gone from her voice. "This could just be anxiety, but we have to be safe. I'll be there in less than fifteen minutes. I swear it."

I hang up, and the paramedics arrive five minutes later, a woman and a man. They look worried when they see me. The woman untangles my arms and begins immediately to take my vitals; the man questions me. Do I know who and where I am? I answer correctly.

She unplugs the stethoscope from her ears and says, "I think her heart rate is one sixty, but it's so fast and irregular I can't be sure."

They exchange troubled looks.

Mary appears in the doorway and introduces herself. "Hi, I'm a friend of hers, I'm the one who called you. We're both first-years at the law school. Is she going to be okay?"

"Ohhh, she's a *law* student," the man says, and smiles with undisguised relief. Both paramedics visibly relax. The woman pats my hand and wraps the blood-pressure flap around my arm, saying, "We get ten or twelve calls a week from either the law school or the medical school, honey. It's almost always anxiety."

She is right.

At the hospital an electrocardiogram and other tests show a sound, healthy heart. I have just experienced my first panic attack, though I have been plagued by numbing anxiety since arriving at the law school. I am given a muscle relaxer to loosen my chest and neck muscles, a prescription for more of the same, and assigned a stress management counselor.

Three hours after we arrive, Mary is still in the ER waiting room, hunched over a textbook lying open in her lap. She is petite with olive skin, green-brown eyes, and brown hair falling straight to the middle of her back. She senses me and looks up as I walk over, her expression a mixture of sadness and relief. It is dark by the time we leave the hospital. It has been snowing all afternoon.

On the drive to my place, Mary tries to console me, "Hell, Lynn, I've felt like having a panic attack myself a couple times this year. Look at me. After Joey killed himself, I started smoking again."

The car skids on the icy road and Mary turns the steering wheel in the direction of the skid, quickly regaining control.

"Hard to believe that was just a few months ago," she says, referring to another first-year--a close mutual friend--hanging himself in a public parking garage during Christmas break.

Mary drops me at Lake Lila Drive. Never has home looked so good, but the air inside is frigid because I turned off the heat during the panic attack. I reset the thermostat at seventy-five, yank off my boots, and aching with exhaustion crawl under the quilts without taking off my coat.

*   *   *

ONE MONTH LATER

When the professor called on Mr. Bradley, I didn't know he was directly to my left until he began to stutter a response to the question on the relationship of assumption of risk theory and contributory negligence. I think Mr. Bradley suffered from allergies, because his nose was always red; that, or he cried a lot. After a split second's wash of relief that the professor hadn't called on me, I was flooded with a new wave of anxiety, realizing that when he finished abusing Bradley, the professor would call on the person sitting on either side of him. Or, he *might* even skip to another row.

I knew the material, but I was terrified of speaking in front of the one hundred person class. I knew if called on my voice would shake, my answers might be shallow and contrived because I couldn't think clearly. My heart was pounding in my ears as I slid my eyes toward the door only a few feet away. I wanted so badly to leave, but my knees were quaking. Taking notes became impossible. I couldn't keep track of what was being said, and my trembling fingers made it impossible to write. When I dropped my pen laughter erupted suddenly. For an instant, I thought the class had seen me drop the pen and was reacting. Then the professor said something else, and the laughter grew bright enough to pierce the fog in my brain.

Mr. Bradley was having trouble!

Now that I paid attention, I could hear the wheeze in his chest

99

as he tried to control his breathing. I could smell the fear rushing from his nostrils and pores, scenting the air with failure and missed opportunity. I could nearly taste his dry-roasted anxiety in the middle of my tongue. I'm ashamed to say this knowledge brought me great joy. It meant the professor would spend more time abusing Bradley, thereby lowering the odds anyone else would be called on that day. That left only tomorrow to worry about. And all the days after that.

I fled to the library after class. After a while my breathing slowed, and my heart stopped racing. My throat unclenched, permitting me to sip ginger ale; the nausea and stomach tremors stopped after that. As anxiety ebbed, contentment flowed in its place, and I couldn't move from that comfortable spot for a long time. I stayed at my carrel for hours, feeling bundled up and secure, as safe and hidden away as the pages of the many texts that surrounded me. Finally, I shrugged on my grey quilted overcoat and felt for my burgundy hat and gloves stuffed in the pockets. I jumbled my four law books, none of which was less than two inches thick, into an oversized shoulder bag, walked down the foot-worn wooden staircase, and exited the main doors of the Legal Research Building. I preferred to study amid the Gothic charms of the old library, instead of in the sleek underground addition completed a few years ago.

I turned left and headed out of the law quad to State Street where my old Mazda hatchback was parked at an expired meter. It began to snow, drifting down in puffy wet flakes, enforcing a muffled quality on the land that was disturbed only by my boots thumping on the pavement. A path had been cleared on the sidewalk, but it was quickly filling in. I used to think that New York winters were bad until I moved to Cheryl Park and the Midwest. The banner across the highway read, "Welcome to the state with four seasons, June, July, August, and Winter." I had thought it was a joke.

Instead of remaining on State and driving toward North Campus and home, I turned right on University, looking for Dino's twenty-four hour Pizza. I was ravenous. I found the eatery and parked at a meter right in front. The wind had picked up, driving the snow sideways into my face, stinging my eyes and making them tear.

Inside, I placed my order at the counter and headed for a corner booth away from the door. Three tables in front were filled with members of the University's basketball team, some of whom I

recognized from watching ABC Sports: four impossibly tall young men-
-three black and one white--whose bent knees reached almost to the
table tops, and a fifth man, white with a cherub's chubby face, who
could only be the coach by the way he dominated their attention. They
watched me pass and we exchanged pleasantries.

The server brought my slices: crisp dense crust, not too much
cheese, lots of mushrooms, just enough onions, and hot enough to burn
my tongue. I finished the first slice quickly and licked salt and tomato
sauce from my fingertips. A swoosh of cold air swept into the room, and
I looked up to see Mary push in the swinging door. She waved to me
before going to the counter to order calzone, coleslaw, and a Coke. By
the time she paid for her food and sat down on the other side of the red-
and-white checkered tablecloth, I'd bolted down the last bite of my
second slice and burped in satisfaction.

Cold air clung to Mary and snuck out of her pockets into the
warmth of the sweet-smelling restaurant. Red smudges of cold frolicked
on her oval face. She was wearing a black wool pea coat which she
proceeded to unbutton. Blue earmuffs and mittens she placed on the
table next to the salt and pepper. Her body language was serious.

"What's the matter with you?" I asked.

"I have disturbing news. Tried to call, but you weren't home.
They posted the moot court judges this afternoon," she said, and waited
for my reaction.

"So?" As usual I didn't know what was going on at the law
school, rarely paying attention to anything outside of class.

She touched my hand with cold fingers and said, "Stabb is
sitting for Fead Club's moot court arguments this year. He's evidently
convinced Professor Ivy to switch with him."

A flash of heat spiked quickly through my chest and my
stomach fluttered. Good thing I'd already eaten. Then followed a
familiar annoyance with myself. What was there to be afraid of, really?

"Think it has anything to do with the petition?" I asked, trying
to be funny and failing.

Mary's mouth turned down and she nodded. "Since he's the
head, make that past-head-thanks-to-you, of the department, I'm sure
he didn't have any problem engineering the switch."

The server brought her order and she began to eat calzone with
a knife and fork, pausing to douse the coleslaw with black pepper.

We both knew what was happening. My petition had forced Stabb to resign as head of the writing and advocacy program. Now he was gunning for me.

My problems with Professor Stabb had started just three months earlier in January of my second semester in law school. He was heavy set, medium height, had pale pebbly skin, small blue eyes, and white hair. A chain smoker in his sixties, he perspired profusely even on the coldest winter days. He was said to be a genius at drafting legislation and had helped write many of the laws enacted by the U.S. Congress in the past thirty years; there was a waiting list each semester for his classes. Incidental to this fame was his role as head of the writing program, which included moot court at the end of the first year: a case already decided, hence moot, would be reargued by pairs of first-years, who had to come through successfully to get to the second year.

Among law professors, teaching is perceived as a divine step above administration. It was only natural then, that Stabb, a celebrity at the law school, would feel that administering the writing program was beneath him. His hands-off approach led to a system where essentially all authority was ceded to twenty-eight "senior judges," third-year students who had complete autonomy to design the curriculum for their individual clubs, assuring there would be no uniformity.

I discovered the down side of the system while researching at the library. Naturally it was snowing, and a strong bitter wind lobbed icy flakes against the window panes. The upper peninsula had been ice-locked for four days, and the National Guard was flying in supplies. I'd already spent eight hours that week working on a writing assignment when a first-year from Darrow Club came in and spent forty-five minutes researching something at the same table where I sat. She was joined by a friend, asking how soon she could break for dinner.

"It's only my writing assignment. Never takes more than an hour," she whispered. "I'll meet you in the lounge in fifteen minutes."

She finished in ten, reshelved her books and left.

I was stunned.

Students in my club spent, say, six hours for the fast workers who knew what they were doing, to ten hours or more for us "thorough" types--every week. Multiply that by twenty or so assignments due the first year, and that amounted to a lot of time. If what I'd heard was true, it meant that some students were being over worked, or some were being under prepared. I shut my books and gathered my things. I was righteously pissed.

For the next few days I talked to first-years from other clubs and discovered that assignments varied from thirty minutes to sixteen hours. I worked my way up the hierarchy complaining first to my senior judge, Tim, in the locker room between classes. Clean cut and preppy with short black hair, grey eyes, and tan-salon coloring, he doubted anything could be done, but said he'd support me.

Next, I met with Professor Stabb in his office, twice. During each meeting he lit a new cigarette every few minutes, using the hot burr of the old one before stubbing it out in an ashtray choked with ashes, butts, chewing gum, and a soiled band-aid. After the first meeting he said he'd think about my ideas and thanked me for coming. The second time he informed me that the current system didn't need fixing.

"As one of my colleagues puts it, there are only about seven great law schools in the United States, and we are consistently ranked in the top of that group. Did you know this year Harvard and Yale tied for first place, and we came in third?" he asked with a smug chuckle, wiping sweat from his forehead with a white handkerchief.

"So you're not willing to make any changes in the program? To regulate the amount of work that's assigned?" I asked.

"No changes are warranted," he said dismissively, flicking ashes with one hand, dragging his handkerchief across the back of his neck with the other. "Sometimes you just get the short end of the stick," he said, referring to my club being among the ones to draw the tougher assignments. "You have to learn to roll with the punches."

Roll with the punches? "Professor Stabb, do you realize we're talking about the loss or gain of up to fifteen hours a week? Does that seem fair to you?"

"Sometimes life isn't fair, Ms. Smith-Capehart. Sometimes circumstances will put you and your client at a disadvantage. You'll have to be able to alter your strategy and succeed with the additional burden."

The brass desk lamp cast a dismal light across the cluttered desk and on to Stabb's loose features. I looked past him out the window where new snow was falling. Then I nodded, said "Okay," and grasped his damp palm before leaving.

The following day I continued my quest: "First-years always

complain about the writing program, but they always manage to make it through, dear," sang my student advisor. The dean of students told me flat out I had to work it out with Stabb. The assistant dean, and Dean Booker himself, said essentially the same thing. The staff were all accessible, polite, and they listened closely before referring me back to Professor Stabb.

I tried to enlist help from the law school student council. I caught up with Ross, another first-year and the newly-elected president, outside the student lounge in Hatcher Hall where classes met. He listened intently and said, "Sure, come to the next meeting. Submit a resolution, I'll second, and we'll open the floor to a discussion on the best ways to proceed." He flashed a hardy smile with perfect teeth. His aqua turtleneck looked as alive as the sea next to his rich black skin. I knew he was sincere, but I couldn't help feeling disappointed. Nothing shorted my fuse faster than conferences and other group discussions. With so much time spent discussing the obvious, the process of obtaining a consensus grated on me.

That night in my apartment I drank freezer-chilled chardonnay while listening to Miles Davis and planning my next step. I turned off all the lights except a blue bulb to match my mood. I thought about my Grandmother and the small war we had waged the summer between fifth and sixth grade. I had decided I wanted to paint the white picket fence that hugged our house and grassy yard. Grand said no, it was too much work for me, and she resisted my nagging for several days before relenting. But once I started, she wouldn't let me stop when I got tired and bored, which was an hour into the job. She told me if I didn't finish I couldn't go to Philadelphia for my two month vacation with cousins.

"It's up to you. Take as long as you want," she said. "But you're not leaving here until that fence is painted."

I whined, cried, pouted, and cajoled, to no effect.

The lesson got clearer with each stroke of the heavy paint brush in my young hand, up and down and up: If you start something you have to finish it. Up and down and up. Up and down and up.

And I could thank Raleigh for my inability to "roll with the punches." My father didn't live to see me enter law school, but throughout my life he encouraged me to, "always question authority," adding that, "the more power it has, the more scrutiny it demands."

So how was I going to change the writing program?

When I decided on a petition I went to Professor Kasilof for advice. He was my criminal law professor with whom I'd developed a mentor relationship. I was one of the few students not intimidated by his status or gruff demeanor and often visited him in his office. He has a brilliant incisive mind and a deeply felt passion for teaching law. If Stabb was a celebrity at the law school, then Kasilof was royalty. He'd been raised in the north Bronx by parents who were Eastern European immigrants, and he harbored an inherent distrust of authority in general and of the police in particular. He taught at Minnesota and Harvard before settling at the University. His passionate writings were cited in *Miranda*, the decision that protects suspects' against self-incrimination, and *Gideon*, the decision that established a suspect's right to be provided with an attorney. *TIME* Magazine once called him "the most overpowering criminal law scholar in the country." He still shows up on 60 Minutes, Today, or Nightline, commenting on euthanasia or the rights of the suspect.

Kasilof was working in his office amid unimaginable clutter, with every surface including the floor piled chest high. When I walked in without an appointment he greeted me and folded his arms high across his lean chest, wearing the wary look of someone expecting trouble. I assumed he'd heard about my other meetings. Fifty-something and basketball tall, with a ruddy complexion and brown hair thinning at the forehead, Kasilof wore glasses on his intelligent face and most of the time dressed like he was color blind. Today he was subdued in gold polyester pants, a green tweed jacket, blue button-down shirt, and brown tie.

He listened patiently without expression as I explained my situation.

"Tell me, is your club among the ones with the heavy work load?" he asked.

"How'd you guess?" I said, and smiled.

"Well," he said in a sharp staccato voice and turned to look quickly out the window. It had been snowing all morning. "What made you decide on a petition for God's sake? Have you tried talking to Hank ... Professor Stabb, about changing the program?"

"I told you I met with him twice. He blew me off. Nicely. They all did. Nothing's going to change unless I do something drastic like circulate a petition. But I don't know how to word it or how many signatures I need to make my point with the law school."

He shook his head and smiled. "You know, Professor Stabb is not going to be happy about this petition."

"I'm not happy about the time I'm spending on legal writing, all because he refuses to properly structure and supervise the program. It's not right."

"You really are fearless aren't you?" he said, blushing slightly, and laughter touched his brown eyes.

I shrugged, thinking it had more to do with a sense of justice. If the people in Fead Club had to do the work, everyone was going to do it.

"Well," he said again, and leaned forward uncrossing his arms, placing both elbows on the desk as he warmed to the task. "You'll need ten to fifteen percent of first-years, that's about three hundred fifty students, so thirty-five to fifty signatures. Petitions usually start with two or three short paragraphs defining the parameters, using the 'whereas, therefore' structure of a contract."

I pulled out a pen, opened my notebook, and hurriedly took notes.

While I circulated the petition--singlehandedly for the first week, traipsing from Hatcher Hall through LRB, to all three underground floors of the new library, and back, for up to ten hours a day--Stabb managed to remain above the fray, only once sending a research assistant to spy on me. By the end of the first week, I'd gathered over a hundred signatures from all three classes, not just first-years. That still didn't seem enough to get anyone's attention, despite what Kasilof had said, but it was taking too long. I hadn't been to class since I'd started this crusade. Mary was supplying me with good notes, but notes could get you only so far. And getting signatures on a petition from law students wasn't easy. Except for my friends who signed without argument, each signature represented five to fifteen minutes while a student read the petition, questioned me about my motives, then debated each point. After all that, some still said no.

I decided to marshal my defenses.

I started by going back to Tim and asking him to write to *The Et Seq*, the law school newspaper, supporting the petition. Since he was part of the system I was attacking, his backing would add credibility. I asked Ross to pass a resolution at the next student council meeting in support of it. (Council minutes were routinely published in the *ES*.) I submitted two articles regarding needed changes, and asked, Alec, another first-year, to submit illustrations accompanying them. I then approached the *ES*, requesting that they run a copy of the petition so everyone would know what it said; that alone could move things along considerably. Rita, the editor-in-chief, volunteered to devote that week's editorial to the issue. Her headline ran, "Sign That Petition." She also coordinated the material so that all the submissions regarding the petition were published in the same weekly issue.

It worked.

After the *ES* was released on Wednesday morning you couldn't go anywhere in the law school without hearing discussions about the petition and the writing program. Second and third-year students got involved even though it was a first-year issue. People who'd previously said no looked for me so they could sign. There was so much interest that I issued copies to other law students who'd volunteered to help. We collected five hundred fifty-one signatures, more than half the student body, and fully seventy-five percent of first-years.

I presented the petition to Assistant Dean Cook, who accepted it with a look of combined respect and disbelief. Six weeks later Professor Stabb resigned and was replaced by a local attorney. Unfortunately, her changes wouldn't be instituted until the following year, but the scrutiny created a more level playing field: longer assignments shrank and shorter ones were expanded, so that all students had more uniform workloads.

After his resignation, Stabb uncaged his animosity. When we passed in the halls he shot me looks that could have uncurled steel wool. I decided not to take any of his classes.

*   *   *

I waited for Mary to finish eating and we walked out together, passing the basketball players who continued to order and eat pizza. They were a bit too enthusiastic and were immediately censured by the coach. Snow flakes continued to whirl frantically in the atmosphere. *Would it never stop?* I couldn't complain about the weather to Mary who grew up in Grand Rapids, Michigan; she would just laugh and look perplexed.

"How much time do I have to prepare and who's my opposition?" I asked.

"You mean besides Professor Stabb," she said, and we both hooted loudly.

"That's not funny," I said, wiping tears from my eyes.

"Sorry. Let's see. You and Peter are facing each other in a zoning action. You represent plaintiff in *Belle Terre v. Boraas*. You argue three weeks from tomorrow. 8:30 p.m."

Back home I realized I hadn't inquired about Mary's case. Feeling awful about a number of things, I tumbled into bed and a fitful sleep peppered with nightmares. At 3:00 a.m. I awoke with a racing heart and my sheets soaked through. After changing the bed linen, I sat up sipping hot cocoa and trying to study for a contracts quiz. Before falling asleep at dawn, I decided to miss class, take a fail on the quiz, and try to make it up on the final.

I climbed wearily out of bed at noon and opened the flannel drapes to soft sunlight falling from an ashen sky. As I stood there it started to snow. I turned away and uttered an obscenity. Hard to believe it was mid April. I went to the refrigerator for tomato juice and vitamins. I'd been taking CoQ10 for a month because I read that it boosted energy. As I urged my morning dose from the bottle, I remembered that it took four to six weeks to begin working. The timing would be fortunate if it worked. I would have greater energy right before moot court.

For the next week, Professor Stabb's switch was the buzz in the hallways. Scores of students, many I didn't know, approached me with supportive comments. It occurred to me that I could sidestep Stabb's transparent offensive by raising objections to the obvious conflict of interest he'd created. The law school administration was generally very lenient, even nurturing, with students. Dean Ruth would simply make other moot court arrangements for me if I requested it. But there were a lot of reasons why I wouldn't run from a confrontation with Stabb: pride, anger, stubbornness. Maybe it was simply a satisfaction I wasn't willing to give him. Even if he demolished my arguments, what would it prove? I'd had eight months of law school. He'd been teaching for thirty years.

The following Monday I was back in class next to Mr. Bradley who was quite relaxed, knowing that only the cruelest professors

108

returned to belittle the same victim in a subsequent class. He knew he was safe for the time being. When my name was called nothing happened, no splash of panic. I answered the question on products liability and added an additional comment on the reading material. My voice was strong and smooth, my breathing regular. I spoke slowly. I couldn't believe it! I was almost sorry when the professor lost interest and moved across the room to ambush Ms. Knox. Almost. It wasn't until summer break, after I'd had the opportunity to experiment, that I was sure CoQ10 was responsible for my new found calm.

I continued to take CoQ10 daily and over the next two weeks I also noted a remarkable increase in my energy. I was able to stay alert no matter how tired I became. But I was most impressed with the inner calm the supplement gave me. It was as though CoQ10 had reset my inner clock, slowed me down, put me in sync with the world. I was able to think better in class, because I wasn't lost in the miasma of fear that usually haunted me. But moot court with Judge Stabb would be the real test.

*   *   *

Peter and I waited outside the small court room on the second floor of Hatcher Hall. We were scheduled to argue last, probably arranged by Stabb, I thought, so he wouldn't have to stick to the ten-minute limitation on questions. I was wearing a severely-cut, navy pin-stripe suit, white silk blouse, navy pantyhose, and two-inch navy high heels. The outfit cost more than the entire rest of the contents of my closet, and I only wore it on legal occasions. Peter's white skin looked pallid next to his black suit, and his cheeks and ears were almost as red as his power tie. He kept running the inside edge of his right palm down over his thick black moustache.

"I feel sick," he muttered. "And I can't remember a f---ing thing."

"Don't worry. It'll all come back to you," I said.

We fell silent and waited.

When I entered the court room, with my high heels clicking sharply against the wood floors—click sway, click sway, click sway, click—I was struck by Stabb's mood, more alive than I'd ever seen him. Tim sat on his left and on his right was Hannah, Tim's junior clerk. All

109

three wore black judicial robes. Tim and Hannah looked worried; they'd both signed the petition. No spectators were allowed, so the court room was empty except for the five of us.

I was excited with anticipation, but not overly nervous when I took the podium first to argue for plaintiff. After a while I realized I was enjoying myself. I spoke for my allotted fifteen minutes. Then Stabb assaulted me with questions for a half hour, but I never faltered. During a pause, Tim leaned over and whispered something in his ear, pointing to his wrist. Stabb looked down at his papers then abruptly told me he had no more questions. I think an urge for a cigarette also helped stop him. For the last few minutes he'd been tapping the index and middle fingers of his right hand against his lips in an unconscious manner that mimicked smoking.

Peter argued well for defendant, but I wasn't paying strict attention. I was too intent on observing Stabb. No longer looking happy, he nearly bristled with irritation and impatience. I don't know what he expected from me that night. I know he didn't get it.

CHAPTER 7

BEE POLLEN AND VITAMIN C COMPLEX
Taken Together In Combination

•Heal And Prevent Colds

•Fight Allergies, Hay Fever, And Sinus Problems--Including Headaches

•Strengthen The Immune System And Improve Resistance

Bee pollen is an almost perfect food containing more protein per gram than meat, eggs, or cheese, as well as an abundance of B vitamins, C vitamins, and Minerals. It consists of tiny fertilized grains collected from flowers by honey bees. Vitamin C Complex contains Vitamin C combined with Rutin, Citrus Bioflavinoids, Hesperidin, and sometimes Acerola. Taken together, Bee Pollen and Vitamin C Complex can have an amazingly curative effect on the immune system, strengthening it and permitting the body to heal or otherwise avoid many common ailments. It is especially helpful in healing and preventing colds, allergies, hay fever, and sinus problems-- including headaches.

Recommended Strength[14]

Bee Pollen--1000 mg

Vitamin C Complex--1000 mg (The dosage strength is for Vitamin C only, the other trace components will be present in varying amounts depending upon the brand.) You may use Vitamin C alone without the other trace elements if you cannot find Vitamin C Complex.

Recommended Form

Bee Pollen--pressed pellet tablets which can be chewed or swallowed

Vitamin C Complex--tablets or capsules

Taken How

A Single Dose: 1 Bee Pollen and 1 Vitamin C Complex (1000 mg each)

A Double Dose: 2 Bee Pollen and 2 Vitamin C Complex (2000 mg each)

A Triple Dose: 3 Bee Pollen and 3 Vitamin C Complex (3000 mg each)

All doses should be taken with eight ounces of juice or other liquids as directed.

---

14 For Bee Pollen the author has had the best results with Puritan's Pride®, Oakdale, NY 11769, (800) 645-1030; and Solgar®, Leonia NJ 07605, (800) 645-2246. Puritan's Pride is available by mail order only. Solgar can be purchased at most health foods stores and sometimes in the health foods section of supermarkets. There are too many quality brands of Vitamin C Complex to mention here. Try to purchase a brand that obtains Vitamin C and other trace elements from rose hips or other food sources. Try to avoid brands that obtain Vitamin C from synthetic ascorbic acid.

Side Effects

None observed with either supplement when taken as directed.

Notes√√

√ Taken alone these supplements will not have the desired therapeutic effect. They should be taken together--at the same time--to be effective as a remedy.

√ Bee Pollen in pressed pellet tablets is used here because of its ease and convenience, as they can be swallowed or chewed. Bee Pollen is also available in a loose pellet form which can be dissolved in hot teas, sprinkled as a topping, and mixed with honey or jam to make a spread. It can also be added to blender drinks.

•Heal And Prevent Colds

1. Take a triple dose of Bee Pollen and Vitamin C Complex at the first signs of a cold.

2. Take a double dose an hour later, and continue every two hours until bedtime.

3. Begin the procedure again the following morning, starting with a triple dose.

4. Continue this daily schedule until your symptoms are gone.

5. Reduce to a double dose three times daily, morning, afternoon, and evening, and continue for three days.

6. At this point you may discontinue the combination or continue to take a single dose twice daily, morning and evening, as a maintenance dose to help prevent colds.

Remedy At A Glance (Bee Pollen And Vitamin C Complex)

	At Onset	One Hour Later	Every Two Hours Until Bedtime
First Day Of Cold And Daily To Relieve Symptoms:	Triple Dose	Double Dose	Double Dose

	Morning	Afternoon	Evening
Daily For Three Days After You Are Better:	Double Dose	Double Dose	Double Dose
Daily As A Maintenance Dose: (Optional)	Single Dose		Single Dose

Notes√√

√ This remedy can make a cold appear to be healed before it really is. For this reason, you should complete all steps of the remedy even if you are feeling better.

√ How do you know whether you have the flu or just a cold? Cold symptoms usually occur from the neck up--sore throat, trouble swallowing, headache, sinus problems, sneezing, stuffy and/or runny nose, watery eyes, and low fever. The primary symptom of the flu is the rapid onset of muscle aches and fatigue. Other flu symptoms can include respiratory inflammation, congestion, runny nose, headache, and high fever. Generally, the flu comes on faster and leaves the person feeling exhausted. Colds come on slower and are less debilitating. See Chapter 4 for more on L-Lysine and how to use it to help heal and prevent flu and other viruses.

√ Certain foods produce mucous in your system and should be avoided or kept to a minimum while treating a cold: (1) all milk products, including ice cream, butter, yogurt, whipped cream, sour cream, etc. (2) all sugar products, especially candy and other sweet desserts, (3) alcohol of any kind.

√ To help heal colds it is recommended that you also take **Echinacea (*only if you do not have an auto-immune disorder*), Beta**

114

Carotene and **Lecithin**. Echinacea greatly stimulates the immune system. Beta Carotene accelerates healing anywhere in the body. Lecithin breaks up mucous to relieve congestion.

Echinacea: Use in 400 mg, capsules only.[15] Take it with eight ounces of juice or other liquids as directed.

1. Take 1600 mg (4 capsules) four times a day, i.e., 8:00 a.m., 1:00 p.m., 6:00 p.m., and 11:00 p.m., and continue until your symptoms are gone.

2. Reduce to 1600 mg (4 capsules) twice a day, morning and evening, and continue for three days.

3. At this point you may discontinue Echinacea or continue to take 800 mg (2 capsules) once a day in the morning, to support a healthy immune system.

4. Remember, do *not* use Echinacea if you have an auto-immune disorder such as rheumatoid arthritis or multiple sclerosis, because stimulating your immune system can worsen your disease and symptoms.

Remedy At A Glance (Echinacea)

	8:00 a.m.	1:00 p.m.	6:00 p.m.	11:00 p.m.
Daily To Relieve Symptoms:	1600 mg	1600 mg	1600 mg	1600 mg

	Morning	Evening		
Daily For Three Days After Your Are Better:	1600 mg	1600 mg		

Daily As A Maintenance Dose (Optional):	800 mg

15 For Echinacea the author has had the best results with Puritan's Pride®, Oakdale, NY 11769, available by mail order only at (800) 645-1030.

See Volume II of this series for more on Echinacea and how to use it to promote a healthy immune system.

Beta Carotene: Use in 25,000 International Units (IU) softgels only. Take it once a day with your largest meal as directed, regardless of the amount you are taking.

1. Take 250,000 IU (10 softgels) daily, beginning on the first day of you cold, and continue for up to five days.

2. If you still have symptoms after the fifth day, reduce to 200,000 IU (8 softgels) daily, and continue at this level until your symptoms are gone.

3. Reduce to 100,000 IU (4 softgels) daily, and continue for three days.

4. At this point you may discontinue Beta Carotene or continue to take 50,000 IU (2 softgels) daily, as a maintenance dose to help keep your respiratory system healthy.

Remedy At A Glance (Beta Carotene)

	Once A Day With Largest Meal
Daily For First Five Days To Relieve Symptoms:	250,000 IU
Daily After Fifth Day To Relieve Symptoms:	200,000 IU
Days For Three Days After You Are Better:	100,000 IU
Daily As A Maintenance Dose: (Optional)	50,000 IU

See Chapter 5 for more on Beta Carotene and how to use it as a remedy to shorten healing time by more than half, and *drastically* reduce wound tenderness and scarring.

Lecithin: Use in 1200 mg softgels only. Take it with eight ounces of juice or other liquids as directed. (Chapter 9 tells you how to use the granular form to supplement your daily doses.)

1. Take 6000 mg (5 softgels) three times daily, morning, afternoon, and evening, beginning on the first day of a cold.

2. Continue at this level as long as you have congestion.

3. Reduce to 6000 mg (5 softgels) twice daily, morning and evening, and continue for three days.

4. At this point you may discontinue Lecithin or continue to take 4800 mg (4 softgels) twice daily, morning and evening, as a maintenance dose to help keep your respiratory system free of congestion.

Remedy At A Glance (Lecithin)

	Morning	Afternoon	Evening
First Day Of Cold And Daily To Relieve Congestion:	6000 mg	6000 mg	6000 mg
Daily For Three Days After You Are Better:	6000 mg		6000 mg
Daily As A Maintenance Dose (Optional):	4800 mg		4800 mg

See Chapter 9 for more on Lecithin and how to use it to help heal arthritis, prevent bloodclot stroke, lower cholesterol, clean out blocked arteries and heart valves without surgery, prevent arteriosclerosis, end gout, and dissolve gallstones.

•Fight Allergies, Hay Fever, And Sinus Problems--Including Headaches

1. Take a triple dose of Bee Pollen and Vitamin C Complex

three times daily, morning, afternoon, and evening, *every day*, whether or not you are experiencing symptoms.

2. During hay fever and allergy season, this dosage may be insufficient to stop your symptoms. At those times, you may take a double dose every two hours as long as you are awake--whatever is necessary to prevent your symptoms.

Remedy At A Glance (Bee Pollen And Vitamin C Complex)

	Morning	Afternoon	Evening
Daily Schedule Generally:	Triple Dose	Triple Dose	Triple Dose
Daily Schedule During Allergy Season:	Every Two Hours Double Dose		

Notes √√

√ To heal any sinus problem it is recommended that you also take **Lecithin**, which breaks up mucous to relieve congestion, pain, and pressure. If you have a sinus *infection*, it is recommended that you also take **Beta Carotene**, which accelerates healing anywhere in the body.

Lecithin: Use in 1200 mg softgels only. Take it with eight ounces of juice or other liquids as directed. (Chapter 9 tells you how to use the granular form to supplement your daily doses.)

1. Take 6000 mg (5 softgels) three times daily, morning, afternoon, and evening, and continue as long as you have any sinus discomfort.

2. Reduce to 6000 mg (5 softgels) twice daily, morning and evening, and continue for one week.

3. Continue to take 4800 mg (4 softgels) twice daily, morning and evening, as a maintenance dose to help keep your sinus free of congestion.

Remedy At A Glance (Lecithin)

	Morning	Afternoon	Evening
Daily To Relieve Congestion:	6000 mg	6000 mg	6000 mg
Daily For One Week After You Are Better:	6000 mg		6000 mg
Daily As A Maintenance Dose:	4800 mg		4800 mg

See Chapter 9 for more on Lecithin and how to use it to help heal arthritis, prevent bloodclot stroke, lower cholesterol, clean out blocked arteries and heart valves without surgery, prevent arteriosclerosis, end gout, and dissolve gallstones.

Beta Carotene: Use in 25,000 IU softgel form only. Take it once a day with your largest meal as directed, regardless of the amount you are taking.

1. Take 250,000 IU (10 softgels) daily for the first two days of each week, i.e., Sunday and Monday.

2. Reduce to 200,000 IU (8 softgels) daily for the next three days, i.e., Tuesday, Wednesday, and Thursday.

3. Reduce to 150,000 IU (6 softgels) daily for the last two days, i.e., Friday and Saturday.

4. Follow this weekly schedule as long as you have any sinus discomfort, then reduce to 100,000 IU (4 softgels) daily, and continue for one week.

5. Continue to take 75,000 (3 softgels) daily, as a maintenance dose to help promote a healthy sinus.

Remedy At A Glance (Beta Carotene)

	Once A Day With Largest Meal		
	Days 1-2	Days 3-5	Days 6-7
Daily To Relieve Symptoms:	250,000 IU	200,000 IU	150,000 IU
Daily For One Week After You Are Better:	100,000 IU		
Daily As A Maintenance Dose:	75,000 IU		

See Chapter 5 for more on Beta Carotene and how to use it as a remedy to shorten healing time by more than half, and *drastically* reduce wound tenderness and scarring.

•Strengthen The Immune System And Improve Resistance

1. Take a single dose of Bee Pollen and Vitamin C Complex twice daily, morning and evening, as a maintenance dose to help promote a healthy immune system and improve your resistance.

Remedy At A Glance (Bee Pollen And Vitamin C Complex)

	Morning	Evening
Daily As A Maintenance Dose:	Single Dose	Single Dose

*   *   *

The following is a case study written as a short story about the man who showed the author how to use Bee Pollen and Vitamin C to stop a cold. Over the years hundreds of others have used this remedy to successfully avoid colds: A willful band of sickly American musicians discovers a cold remedy, while touring European clubs guided by a repressed but loveable French agent.

"Flight From Destiny"

Robert Eznik was the first Frenchman I knew personally. He was unkind to no one, but he was continually abused by those closest to him. And I've never observed a man so accepting of misuse. He was a durable victim, reverting quickly to original form no matter how badly he was bent, folded, or spindled.

Robert was five feet, six inches tall, medium weight, with a hawk-like nose, and a beaten-down demeanor that made him appear older than his thirty-five years. His mother was French, his father Turkish, and he was a man of contradictions: Neatly combed and oiled brown hair did not settle with the sprinkle of dandruff that never left his rounded shoulders. The playful sparkle in his dark chocolate eyes belied the pallor of his fleshy face when he smiled, which was often, a smile that seemed always on the verge of laughter. He was said to be very shrewd with numbers, a CPA, but he worked as an agent traveling through western Europe with his only act, J.J. & Sam. He came from "money," but during our six month business relationship he wore only a badly frayed black suit, always with a white dress shirt similarly frayed, narrow black tie, black hose and wing-tips. Black wool scarf and leather gloves were sometimes included, but no overcoat even in winter.

When in Paris, Robert lived in his mother's apartment off the Champs Elysees, and rarely spoke to his father, whom his mother loathed. I met her once. She was several inches taller than her only son and stick narrow. Long white hair was swept on top of her head in a loose knot secured with an ornate jeweled comb studded with stones that appeared genuine. Her face was bare of cosmetics, giving her translucent skin a slightly blue cast. She wore a black taffeta dress with a lace hem topping her ankles. A white silk scarf was around her neck.

Robert introduced us, and she looked through me, her features unyielding, neck stiff, without responding to my polite, "Bonjour, Madame Eznik." He apologized while she continued to stare at a point over my left shoulder. It wasn't me, he said, she treated all his friends that way, because they were *his* friends.

Their ten room apartment was well appointed but smelled of loneliness. In Robert's walk-in closet, there was hanging only a single change of clothes identical to the black suit ensemble he wore everyday;

spare black hose sat alone on a shelf.

He saw the look on my face and said, "Madame burned my clothes, all except these." The flourish of his gesture took in what he was wearing and the items in the closet. "She was angry at my father at the time, because ... well, they were arguing long distance, and he hung up on her."

Madame was also a vegetarian who permitted her son to consume only steak cooked medium rare, potatoes, and red wine. When someone asked Robert why she wanted him to eat meat when she didn't, he smiled and said, "I do not know. Perhaps she is trying to kill me."

Robert wanted to make a good impression on our band, Flight From Destiny. It was our first gig, and his first chance to portray a new, less fallible self, but all he could do now was cast his glance away, trying to conceal his embarrassment, trying to react in a way that said what was happening wasn't as bad as it looked. The burly club owner, taller by fully two heads, leaned close into Robert's face as he berated him, punctuating groups of words by slamming his open palm into the smaller man's chest. Each blow danced Robert backward, closer to the half-wall separating the lobby from the bar and dance floor. The owner's long unruly hair swished anxiously over his forehead and around his shoulders. I spoke no French, but no language skills were necessary to interpret Long Hair's rage. We were late--Robert had been showing us the city--but I didn't think that could be the source of so much anger. Robert responded to the assault in small apologetic murmurings, neck craned forward staring at Long Hair's feet. His gaze floated as high as the open shirt collar exposing a monkey chest of hair, before surrendering to the feet again.

Tension spawned in my stomach as I watched. "How much of this s--- are we going to let Robert take before we help him?" I asked the six musicians gathered behind me.

"Whoa baby, slow down. I'm sure the man knows what he's doing." Cole said. At twenty-three he was the oldest and the band leader. "We just met this guy," he said, and came to stand close to me, placing his trumpet case on the floor and hugging me to his lanky body. We had met our freshman year in college and had been living together for three years since we dropped out of school. He was a tall, striking black man with buttermilk skin, light-brown eyes looking out of thick horn-rimmed glasses, and a remarkable widow's peak topping his forehead. A native New Yorker, he had been a child prodigy, played four instruments, and composed.

At twenty-one I wasn't sure what I wanted to do, but one of my favorite games as a child had been playing "office," so I agreed to be the band's business manager. I enjoyed the company of musicians and other show people--they had many faults and were often self-centered, but their spirits were generous and their hearts free of prejudice--and I had too much ego to be a groupie.

"You'd better listen to your man and just stay out of it," Mark said, backing Cole up as usual. He placed his tenor saxophone case vertically on the floor and carefully seated himself on top of it, balancing his feet on either side. He was tall and moved with deliberate slowness, shoulders hunched, even when in a hurry. An easy going farm boy from Iowa who'd practiced afternoons in an unheated barn with peeling red paint, Mark saw life in simple terms. He'd come to The Big Apple to be a professional musician; after just a year he was touring Europe. In his mind he'd already made it. His left hand strayed to his chin where he began to pick absently at a new pimple, while he watched Long Hair manhandle Robert. Numerous pea shapes marred the brown skin on his neck and lower jaw.

"I ain't goin' to risk my life for no honky, 'dat's for sure," Hal said, in a voice as high as a woman's and deeply seasoned with Jamaican patois. Seated at a glass-top table, he was tapping out rhythms with the drum sticks he always carried in his right back pocket. Ta-ta, ta-ta-ta, ta-ta; ta-ta, ta-ta-ta, ta-ta. Tall, hyperactive and handsome, he had a Julliard degree and classical training like Cole. "Anyway, 'dat club owner look like he can kick him some serious a--."

"So you're saying if Robert were black, you'd help him? You're unbelievable, man. If he were black you'd think up another reason not to fight, 'cause you're a wuss. Got nothing to do with racial pride." That came from Ralph the bass player. Bear shaped and chubby soft, with a big afro, deep black skin, extra spaces between small front teeth, and a gentle nurturing manner, he prided himself on being unrelentingly color-blind.

"I tell you what. Your a-- is black enough." Ta-ta, ta-ta-ta, ta-ta. "Go 'head ova' 'dere and see if I come help *you*." Turning to Jim, Hal added, "You a honky boy so why you don't go ova' 'dere 'an help your brudder?"

"Screw you. Ain't no damn honky, I'm Italian," Jim said, and drops of laughter pattered through the group. Seated across from Hal, he was playing finger piano on the same table top. Born and raised in the northeast Bronx next door to Ralph, Jim was jockey-sized with long sandy-brown hair. He had blue eyes set in a pixie-like face with a long, upturned nose, and a mere slash for a mouth. At nineteen he was the youngest and my right-hand man; I couldn't imagine managing those animals without him to help me ride herd. He drove the vehicles, supervised set-up and break-down, and cared lovingly for all the equipment, including the sound system which was his. He also produced other assorted small miracles whenever I requested them. "But maybe she's right," he said, and stopped with his fingers in mid air spelling out a C-chord over major ninth.

"Some f---ed up way to run a tour," Julian said, causing us to turn and look at him. He had joined the group for this tour and was considered as much of a newbie as Robert. An East Hampton rich boy who dressed in second-hand clothes, he replaced our regular guitarist (also named Julian), when he refused to leave his girlfriend for the tour. This Julian had already taken a major step in the wrong direction, letting it out that he didn't really need the money, just wanted the experience. Squarely built with sharp features in a pale homely face, his thin brown hair always looked uncombed and his blue eyes ill-tempered.

Under his breath, Jim muttered, "Now there's your honky."

"What about it?" I asked again. Robert was slowly folding in on himself to ward off the blows to his chest. "He's one of us now, we should help him."

"I love the way she say *we*." Ta-ta, ta-ta-ta, ta-ta. "Like she actually goin' to be doin' some of the fightin' if we do go ova' 'dere. "

"Maybe this is the way they do business over here," Cole offered.

I started across the floor while the thought was still forming that what was happening would last until it was over, that Robert wouldn't end it, that even if he could take it, I couldn't.

When I reached the two men my heart was pounding in my ears. I shouted at Long Hair to stop and punched the arm holding Robert's lapel. Both men stopped and turned to look at me, incredulous for several seconds. Long Hair was breathing deeply, thickening the air with garlic scent; Robert's breathing was slow and regular. When Long Hair let go of the lapel and turned to face me, he looked amused and more than a little turned on. He dropped his gaze down my body and back up, saying something lewd in French, before noticing the movement behind me. The musicians, except Julian, had followed me across the room, and now stepped between us. None of them was a genuine tough guy, so they had to improvise the walk-it-talk-it of the street. They were good enough to convince Long Hair, who held up his hands, palms facing out in a gesture of compromise. He said something to Robert, his tone low and sinister, and stalked across the dance floor and up the red carpeted stairs to his office.

"Hurry, hurry. We must hurry and set up," Robert said, obviously relieved. "We have only twenty minutes before the doors open."

The first two sets were flawless. Cole opened each with the classical, "Also Sprachen" theme from *2001*, which was an attention grabber with its slow theatrical buildup. It also helped that patrons couldn't dance to it and had to wait for what would come next--which would be hot-buttered Motown funk or James Brown, followed by Chicago or the Rolling Stones. By then the dancers were sweaty and Cole cooled them down with his sweet flute, gave them a chance to rub bellies with a ballad from the Carpenters or Patti LaBelle. For ballads, Hal put his sticks in his back pocket and used brushes. Once each set they played one of Cole's originals.

During the third set, Long Hair slipped quietly into a chair at the table where Robert and I sat talking and drinking wine. His English wasn't as smooth as our agent's, but I could understand him. He ordered more wine for us, praised the band, apologized for losing his temper, lifted my left hand from the table and kissed it. Still holding my hand, he told me not to worry about what I'd seen. He punched Robert's arm and laughed when he winced. I retrieved my hand. All was forgiven. Until smoke appeared on stage behind Flight From Destiny's wall of electronic equipment.

Robert glanced at me with a hopeful look that said, Please tell me this is part of the show. The audience applauded. The musicians kept their expressions carefully zipped. All I could think was, if being late sent Long Hair into yellow delirium, what would he do if we started a fire on stage. So far it was only smoke, but.... Long Hair didn't notice when Robert excused himself to go to the bathroom, so absorbed was he with the action on stage. He frowned and squinted, uncertain, as exotic fingers of smoke gestured to the dancers, still not sure it wasn't part of the act. *Didn't the Americans have special equipment?*

Jim reacted first, leaving the Hammond to fiddle with the wiring. On the floor the dancers were slowing, noticing the hole left by the organ's departure and the biting smell of burning wire. Jim unplugged the microphones, shrinking the vocals. Long Hair stood slowly, recognition dawning. I began searching for something at the bottom of my handbag. The band played on.

Long Hair tore past my chair nearly toppling me, winging toward the stage, screaming what I imagined were French obscenities-- the only word I understood was "Eznik". He reached the stage and jumped up, dove past the horn players, grabbed one of the smoking speakers, unplugged it, and dragged it to the dance floor, away from the velvet stage curtains. Why'd he do that, I thought, as I crossed my arms and sighed deeply, waiting for Jim's reaction. He paused one-two-three-four seconds for Long Hair to set his beloved speaker down with a thud on the dance floor. Then Jim leaped silently onto his back, straddling Long Hair's waist, jockey-like, left arm around his neck, right fist entwined in the owner's indignant locks.

The instant Jim jumped on Long Hair they became the center of the universe, and all matter converged on them: The bartender whizzed from behind the bar. Two bouncers at the bottom of the wide staircase lumbered over. Patrons fled tables to get closer to the action. Flight From Destiny left the stage in a flash to unsaddle Long Hair and retrieve Jim before he could get hurt. Ralph plucked him off and carried him under one arm back to the stage. Jim regained his composure immediately when Ralph put him down--I'm not sure he ever lost it-- and returned to his ailing equipment. But I didn't know if Long Hair would ever be the same; he looked dazed and broken as he stumbled past me and up the stairs to his office.

Cole, Mark, and Hal sat down at the table, and we watched the bouncers urge customers upstairs to the exit; Ralph stayed on stage to help Jim; Julian went outside to buy chewing gum.

I started laughing not because it was funny, but because it was ridiculous. The others watched me in amazement. I was doubled over the table, sucking for air, wiping tears from my eyes. Trying to stop only made it worse. "I'm sorry," I gasped, feeling lightheaded. I was still jet-lagged and hadn't eaten a real meal since I'd left the United States four days earlier.

"You think it's funny we just burned out the alternator and can't use our electrical equipment?" Cole asked. He was referring to our equipment brought from the United States that needed only one hundred twenty volts, while the French electrical system ran on two hundred twenty volts. Without an alternator to vary the current, too much electricity would come through the line and damage the equipment within minutes. I was laughing too hard to speak and could only shake my head. They resisted my mood as long as they could before giving up to laughter.

Ralph arrived at the table followed shortly by Jim, whose face and hands were smudged with soot. "The alternator's finished," he said, unnecessarily, looking like he wanted to cry. "We're f---ed." We studied him quietly for an instant before laughter burst free again. Jim didn't think it was funny, but the rest of us laughed until our ribs were exhausted and our cheeks ached.

Robert was waiting in the ten-passenger mini bus we were using on the tour, a silver Mercedes. Without getting out he motioned for us to hurry. I got on the bus and we greeted each other without saying anything more. I took a seat in the last row. I didn't know what to say to him, and he kept his head angled away from me, watching the club entrance while the men loaded. I was glad he'd bailed on us but disturbed by it at the same time. If he had stayed he would have been an easy target for Long Hair. On the other hand, by leaving--after getting us there late--Robert had not made a good showing. It is the agent who is supposed to come to the defense of the client.

Safe at home in New York City I hadn't realized how completely we would depend on him while in Europe. He arranged everything except where and when we ate. We knew the names of the clubs, but not the countries they were in or how to get there. I had an itinerary that was meaningless without him. And none of us spoke a second language.

My discomfort was heightened by guilt: Robert and I had met at an audition in New York four weeks earlier on November 1. Flight From Destiny was trying out for house band at a dance club on west 52nd Street; Robert was looking for a back up band for J.J. & Sam.

Their original band quit in the middle of the tour with fourteen weeks left on the schedule. If I had been older or wiser I'd have asked why. (Musicians in our strata didn't walk away from fourteen weeks of work.) Instead, all I heard was that he was offering us a free trip to Europe. I committed Flight From Destiny on the spot, even though it meant our singer, Tesha, couldn't come with us. Worse, in my haste to secure the job, I failed to get the return tickets up front. Robert express-mailed seven *one-way* plane tickets from New York to Brussels; we would drive from there to Paris. I was so happy I accepted his weak explanation: "Why should I spend money for return tickets now, when you will not need them for three months?"

By the time we left Paris the next morning driving southeast toward Dijon, the men were all complaining of cold symptoms. The stress of the trip from New York and the recent events had lowered everyone's resistance. When we pulled out of Auxerre, after stopping for petrol and sandwiches, everyone but Robert and I was displaying the usual symptoms. I was riding in the first seat behind Jim who was driving, half-reading an English version of *Avant Garde* Magazine and half-watching the French countryside race by. All around me were intermittent sounds of sneezing, coughing, and noses being emptied of mucous. It was positively rhythmic. Directly behind me, Hal provided a percussive rondo as he hacked phlegm into a handkerchief. They were a malefic symphony.

I was huddled against the window, nestled in with a pillow and red blanket with TWA monogrammed in large blue letters, trying desperately to keep my back to the infestation. A crescendo of sneezes and coughs rang out, and I burrowed deeper.

It had taken Robert several hours to acquire a new alternator, which task he pursued single-mindedly. His actions went a long way in redeeming him in the eyes of the musicians, especially Jim. Robert was asleep now, serene in the seat beside me. Cole and Mark were studying sheet music across the aisle. Robert's head lolled against the seat back moving in a slight rhythm that matched the bus's motion. His jaw was collapsed open. He didn't wake up when Julian sneezed directly into his face, while standing to stretch his legs.

"Cover your mouth you disgusting slob," I yelled, and pulled the blanket over my ears.

I stared out the window at the blur of

countrysidegreenskyblucloudwhitemountaingreybrickredandhighway black whizzing past, and thought about the upcoming tour. After Dijon, we would meet J.J. & Sam--both black Americans--in Geneva and open a concert with them, then continue southeast to Turin to begin a one month tour through Italy. I wondered how the band would get along with the singers, a Sam & Dave knock-off act, and how they got along with Robert. I didn't know that coming between our agent and the assorted bullies in his life would become an everyday occurrence.

It was two in the afternoon when we spilled out of the bus in front of Club Toulouse. The musicians were tired and sick but had to unpack equipment and set up before they checked into their rooms. Robert and I would walk directly to the hotel a few blocks away; the band would come over after they set up. This arrangement was fine with me. I couldn't wait to see a bed and lay down. My temples and the top of my head were pounding. My throat was raw-sore, making every breath uncomfortable. A tickling in my throat put water in my eyes and caused me to cough irregularly. My nose was both stopped up and runny, making it difficult to sniff back the watery stream that threatened my upper lip.

As we walked the narrow streets, I gazed at fast moving snow clouds threatening in an overcast sky, thinking that it wasn't cold enough for snow. The streets were filled with people on their way home for the traditional two-hour lunch, most carrying bunches of red, yellow, orange, or purple flowers, with two-foot baguettes jutting from the crook of an arm. Robert took my elbow to stop me and pointed to a small hotel two doors down. "That is where we are staying. And you and Cole have a room on a separate floor as you requested." He steered me down a side street away from the hotel, saying, "But first I want to take you to get something for your cold."

"Where are you taking me?" I asked, unable to hide my annoyance at being sick.

Robert urged me forward gently. "This will take only a few minutes. It is very close."

The herbalist's store was tucked in the corner of a covered street. Pungent aromas of spices, dried flowers, and crushed leaves floated out the door each time it was opened and remained trapped in the confined space. No exterior sign was necessary and none appeared. The store's presence was inescapable, even to a stuffy nose, almost from the moment you turned into the street. The effect was overwhelming but pleasant. My throat eased the minute I entered the warm shop out of the damp wintry air.

Inside, the herbalist sat facing the door on a bench behind a long table. He was grinding lavender colored flowers in a stone pestle and mortar and periodically adding bits of a fine yellowish powder and more lavender flowers. The shop was comfortably warm and dimly lighted--except for a bright spotlight illuminating where the herbalist worked--aiding the tranquil atmosphere. A Dave Brubeck album was playing in a back room behind a beaded curtain. The wood walls were stained dark brown and were completely obscured in spots by hanging herbs. While Robert talked to the herbalist, I circled the periphery of the room, looking into wooden barrels and large glass jars, that had white cards attached to clear plastic lids describing their contents.

The herbalist had silver hair and grey eyes. He was fair complected with a thick white moustache that sectioned his long, narrow face into unequal halves. He rose and went to the back of the store through the beaded curtain, emerging with a large round jar. He opened it and carefully scooped some of the contents into two brown cloth bags with tie strings at the top. He filled the bags and tied them securely. He also gave us a jar of jasmine honey. Robert paid him fifty francs. While I waited for them to complete the transaction, I opened one of the bags containing fresh bee pollen granules--tiny kernels that still held the faint colors of their birth flowers. Reds and pale blues were there, yellow predominated; the fragrance was chalky sweet.

"What am I supposed to do with this, Robert?" I asked as soon as we were outside, not bothering to hide my scepticism, then sneezed several times in succession when the cold air struck my inflamed membranes.

"My name is pronounced Row-bear," he said, in a pained voice. "Every hour you must take a tablespoon each of bee pollen and honey mixed in hot water as a tea. Drink it fast. Begin as soon as you take a hot-hot shower."

"Do we have a private bath in our room here?" I asked, and blew my nose in a tissue.

"No, of course not. But at this time of day no one will be using the public shower."

"Well, how long do I have to take the bee pollen?"

"For as long as you have the cold, and then for two days more."

"Uumph," I said, unconvinced. "What's it supposed to do, *Rowbear*?"

"It will strengthen your immune system and make it impossible for the cold to remain in your body. But you must take it exactly as I have told to you."

"Are you going to take it?" I wasn't swallowing anything before he did.

"*Pardone-moi*? You think I am trying to poison you?"

I didn't answer. He took one of the herbalist's bags from me and opened it. While holding one side, he tilted the bag to pour a handful which he scooped into his mouth. I could hear the crunch of the pollen while he chewed. He smiled when I poured my own handful and tossed it into my mouth.

I made a face. "Yeccch."

"*Ah, oui*, that is why it is better with honey in tea."

"Thought you only ate steak, potatoes, and red wine."

"*Oui, habituellement.* But sometimes I eat more. I am very fond of licorice, for instance, but Madame does not know that," he said, and flashed me a look of uncertainty.

It was difficult getting hot water every hour to make tea, so I began eating the bee pollen by the spoonful and washing it down with tangerine slices. Within four hours my sore throat and other symptoms were waning, and I continued to feel better throughout the evening. The next morning I was symptom free and forgot about the bee pollen. All day I bragged about getting over the cold quickly and tried unsuccessfully to convince the musicians to try the same remedy. By dinner time I was sick again. This time my symptoms were far worse and included chills and fever, as though the cold bacteria were angry at me for disrupting their breeding cycle.

Cole was working on a song he was writing for me called, "Sundown," my favorite time of day, when Ralph and Jim stopped by to remind him they were due at the club for rehearsal. I stayed in bed after he left, dozing, until I heard someone peck at my door. It was Robert, carrying a large plastic shopping bag and a silver coffee pot of steamy hot water. I let him in and climbed back under the covers, reaching for another tissue to blow my nose.

"In case you are having trouble getting hot water for your tea," he said, and set the coffee pot on the small nightstand. He tossed the plastic shopping bag on the bed. Inside were more tissues, bee pollen, honey, tangerines, six croissants, and two thick wool blankets, both forest green. I opened the blankets and spread them across the bed one atop the other.

"Thank you," I murmured, truly grateful. "What about the guys? Are you giving them extra blankets too?"

"*Certainement*. If they wish it." Robert said, and proceeded to scold me for not following his instructions. He repeated them and this time I listened: Every hour, plus two days more after I felt better.

Robert sat down in the small armchair next to the bed. He sat quietly for several minutes while I enjoyed the growing heat being trapped by the heavy, double layer of wool. I was about ready to purr. He scratched his scalp then smoothed the hair back in place and examined his fingernails. He cleared his throat and opened his mouth to speak, blushed to his scalp and closed his mouth again without speaking.

"What's the matter?" I asked, biting down on a tangerine section, the sweet juice making the corners of my jaw burn with pleasure.

"I want to apologize. I should not have left you the other night. I am sorry." Once I uncorked him he poured smoothly. "Sometimes I can be very stupid, very cowardly. I promise I will not leave you alone in a crisis again. I know I am responsible for all of you while you are here. I will not forget again."

I didn't know if I could believe him, but it was certainly what I wanted to hear.

As it turned out, Robert kept his word ... most of the time. And the bee pollen remedy worked as he promised when I took it correctly. It was hard to remember to take it when I didn't feel bad, but I managed. I tried to share the information with the band. Somehow their artistic sensibilities were put off by the knowledge that bees secrete a substance on pollen to make it sticky, so they won't drop it during the trip back to the hive. This squeamish outlook seemed odd coming from men who'd eaten hog-testicle sausages with their eggs every morning that week. They refused the remedy and remained ill, sneezing and coughing for three weeks more, through Dijon into Turin and Milan, as the cold circled the band twice like a sustained coda, before it left.

132

CHAPTER 8

ACIDOPHILUS

•Stop Yeast Infections And Feminine Itching
Relieving Discomfort Within Hours And Sometimes Minutes

•Help Prevent Diarrhea
Avoiding "Traveler's Diarrhea"
Getting Rid Of Diarrhea Generally

•Fight Colon Cancer, Crohn's Disease, And Other Intestinal Disorders
Promoting A Healthy Intestinal Tract

•Restore Your Intestinal Balance When Taking Antibiotics
Avoiding Diarrhea, Constipation, And Other Intestinal Reactions

•Get Rid Of Ugly Toenail Fungus
Stopping Toenails From Thickening And Getting Dark

Acidophilus is a live lactobacillus, one of the friendly germs present in a healthy intestinal tract and other vital areas. Used topically and internally as directed, it is a safe effective way to eliminate numerous conditions. And at approximately five cents per dose or application, you can't beat the price. Think of a yeast infection, diarrhea or other intestinal disorders as a battle between intruder microbes and the friendly family of bacteria that inhabits your body--your tenant bacteria, so to speak. These conditions occur when the foreign microbes outnumber your friendly bacteria and cause an imbalance. Adding Acidophilus to your diet introduces millions of friendly bacteria that combat the foreign microbes upon contact.

For example, Acidophilus can stop a yeast infection and its symptoms, bringing remarkable relief, sometimes within a few minutes of topical application. The pH starts moving toward a healthier balance as soon as it is applied. Some women experience immediate relief and need only one or two applications to end a yeast infection. For others, healing can take from several hours to a few days, depending upon the severity of the infection.

Acidophilus can also be effective for treating intestinal disorders such as diarrhea, and, when used in combination with other supplements, Crohn's disease, inflammatory bowel disease and colon cancer. It can restore your intestinal balance when taking antibiotics (antibiotics kill all bacteria, including the "good" ones you need to promote health, which is why many women get yeast infections when using them). It can prevent toenail fungus and thick discolored toenails. It is also recommended as a general precaution against diarrhea and other intestinal disorders sometimes experienced when traveling to foreign countries.

Recommended Strength[16]

Use a formula containing active Lactobacillus Acidophilus, measured in the millions.

Recommended Form

Orally: Softgels or capsules

Topically: Softgels *only*

---

[16] There are only one or two companies that sell Acidophilus in softgels, the best form for topical use, which works equally well for oral use. The author has had the best results with Puritan's Pride® softgels, Oakdale, NY 11769, (800) 645-1030, available by mail order only.

Used How

Orally: Take it on an empty stomach whenever possible; take it with eight ounces of juice or other liquids as directed.

Topically: Wash your hands, and snip the top off one or more softgels with scissors. For yeast infections and vaginal itching, squeeze the contents onto a fingertip and apply liberally around the vaginal area as directed. For use on toenail fungus, you may squeeze the contents directly on to the infected toenails.

Side Effects

None observed when taken and used as directed. *But*, be sure not to exceed the recommended *oral* amounts. Topically, you can use as much Acidophilus as you need, but too much taken orally can cause an imbalance in one of the other families of friendly bacteria. If this occurs you can be very vulnerable to infection and may need antibiotics to rebalance your system. This may also occur if you purchase a brand with lactobacillus measured in the "billions," instead of the "millions" as recommended.

Notes√√

√ Acidophilus gel is essentially odorless, but when used topically it can leave a slightly oily, yellow residue which over time stains cloth. It is recommended that you wear a panty liner if you are using it as a remedy for yeast infection. When using it as a topical remedy for toenail fungus, it can turn the toes of white socks a dirty yellow.

•Stop Yeast Infections And Feminine Itching

Relieving Discomfort Within Hours And Sometimes Minutes

(Acidophilus Topically)

1. Wash the external vaginal area thoroughly but gently with a mild soap and lukewarm water before your first application of the day. You may apply Acidophilus as often as you wish. Remember, you will need softgels for topical use.

2. Use the contents of one or more softgels applied around the outside of the vagina and inside the opening as far as your finger can penetrate. Use as many softgels as necessary to bring temporary relief.

3. You can feel better within a minute or two of application, but the symptoms may return several hours or even minutes later. Repeat the application as often as necessary to bring temporary relief.

4. When your symptoms are gone, continue the procedure once a day for three days.

Remedy At A Glance (Acidophilus Topically)

	As Often As Necessary
Apply To Vaginal Area To Relieve Symptoms:	One or More Softgels
	Once A Day
Apply For Three Days After You Are Better:	One Softgel

Notes√√

√ The symptoms of a yeast infection might also be indications of a more serious condition which may require *immediate medical attention*. This remedy is designed for women who know they have a

136

yeast infection.

√ While the itching and burning discomfort can be alleviated quickly, if you are also experiencing an abnormal discharge, continue the topical applications until that too disappears.

√ If you experience chronic yeast infections, it is recommended that you also take **Acidophilus** orally to help balance your system.

(Acidophilus Orally)

1. Take two softgels or capsules once a day in the morning, and continue for one week.

2. Reduce to one softgel or capsule daily, and continue for one week.

3. Reduce to one softgel or capsule every other day, and continue for two weeks.

4. At this point, *stop taking Acidophilus orally*, until you detect another deficiency.

Remedy At A Glance (Acidophilus Orally)

	Mornings
Daily For One Week To Relieve Symptoms:	Two Softgels or Capsules
Daily For One Week To Relieve Symptoms:	One Softgel or Capsule
Every Other Day For Two Weeks To Relieve Symptoms:	One Softgel or Capsule

Maintenance Dose Not Recommended

•Help Prevent Diarrhea

Avoiding "Traveler's Diarrhea"

(Acidophilus Orally)

1. Take one softgel or capsule, once a day in the morning.

2. Begin the treatment three days before you leave on your trip, and continue through your first two days back home.

3. At this point, *stop taking Acidophilus orally*, until you take another trip.

Remedy At A Glance (Acidophilus Orally)

	Mornings
Daily Beginning Three Days Before Your Trip:	One Softgel or Capsule
Daily While Traveling To Foreign Country:	One Softgel or Capsule
Daily For First Two Days Back Home:	One Softgel or Capsule

Maintenance Dose Not Recommended

Getting Rid Of Diarrhea Generally

(Acidophilus Orally)

1. Take four Acidophilus softgels or capsules at onset, and repeat every three hours until your symptoms are gone.

2. Reduce to one softgel daily in the morning, and continue for three days.

3. At this point *stop taking Acidophilus orally*, until you

experience diarrhea again.

Remedy At A Glance (Acidophilus Orally)

	Every Three Hours
Daily To Relieve Symptoms:	Four Softgels or Capsules

	Mornings
Daily For Three Days After You Are Better:	One Softgel or Capsule

Maintenance Dose Not Recommended

•Fight Colon Cancer, Crohn's Disease, And Other Intestinal Disorders

Promoting A Healthy Intestinal Tract

(Acidophilus Orally)

1. Take two softgels or capsules once a day in the morning, and continue for two weeks.

2. Reduce to one softgel or capsule daily, and continue for four weeks.

3. Reduce to one softgel or capsule every other day, and continue, as a maintenance dose to help promote a healthy intestinal tract.

4. When using a maintenance dose, *stop taking Acidophilus orally, for one week each month* to avoid an imbalance in your system.

Remedy At A Glance (Acidophilus Orally)

<u>Mornings</u>

Daily For Two Weeks
To Relieve Symptoms: Two Softgels or Capsules

Daily For Four Weeks
To Relieve Symptoms: One Softgel or Capsule

Every Other Day As A
Maintenance Dose: One Softgel or Capsule

<u>Remember To Stop For One Week Each Month During Long-Term Use</u>

•Restore Your Intestinal Balance When Taking Antibiotics

Avoiding Diarrhea, Constipation, And Other Intestinal Reactions

(Acidophilus Orally)

1. Starting half-way through your antibiotic regimen--or as soon as you detect symptoms of an imbalance--take two softgels or capsules once a day, in-between doses of antibiotics.

2. Continue at this level until you have completed the antibiotics.

3. Reduce to one softgel or capsule every day in the morning, and continue for one week.

4. Reduce to one softgel or capsule every other day in the morning, and continue for one week.

5. At this point, *stop taking Acidophilus orally*.

Remedy At A Glance (Acidophilus Orally)

	When You Detect Symptoms Or Half-way Through Antibiotic Regimen
Daily To Relieve Symptoms:	Two Softgels or Capsules
Daily For One Week After You Are Better:	One Softgel or Capsule
Every Other Day For One Week After You Are Better:	One Softgel or Capsule

Maintenance Dose Not Recommended

•Get Rid Of Ugly Toenail Fungus

Stopping Toenails From Thickening And Getting Dark

(Acidophilus Topically)

1. Wash your feet thoroughly with soap and warm water before your first application of the day. Make sure your feet and toenails are completely dry before applying Acidophilus. You may apply it as often as you wish. Remember, you will need softgels for topical use.

2. Apply the contents of one or more softgels directly to the infected toenails, along all four sides and across the face. Generally, one softgel contains enough applications for several toenails, but use as many as you need.

3. Put on a pair of socks, being careful to avoid wiping off the gel. You do not have to wear socks after the application, but the oily gel will attract dust, hairs, and other detritus.

4. Cut your infected toenails after one week of daily Acidophilus applications. Keep them as short as possible for the duration of the treatment. At least once a week cut away the thick skin that accumulates in the corners and on the sides of infected toenails. If

141

possible, leave your toenails unpainted for the first three weeks of topical use.

5. It can take a very long time--up to a year or more--before your toenail returns to a substantially healthy state. But the difference in the toenail can be remarkable as it improves, growing out thinner, softer, and lighter in color.

Remedy At A Glance (Acidophilus Topically)

Apply To Toenails Daily To Relieve Symptoms:	After Washing And Drying Feet
	One Or More Softgels

Notes√√

√ When you begin the remedy, it is recommended that you also take **Acidophilus** orally to enhance healing.

(Acidophilus Orally)

1. Take two softgels or capsules once a day in the morning, and continue for two weeks.

2. Reduce to one softgel or capsule once a day in the morning, and continue for four weeks.

3. Reduce to one softgel or capsule every other day, and continue as a maintenance dose until your symptoms are gone.

4. When using a maintenance dose, *stop taking Acidophilus orally, for one week each month* to avoid an imbalance in your system.

5. When your symptoms are gone, *stop taking Acidophilus orally*, until you detect toenail fungus again.

Remedy At A Glance (Acidophilus Orally)

	Mornings
Daily For Two Weeks To Relieve Symptoms:	Two Softgels or Capsules
Daily For Four Weeks To Relieve Symptoms:	One Softgel or Capsule
Every Other Day As A Maintenance Dose:	One Softgel or Capsule

Remember To Stop For One Week Each Month During Long-Term Use

---

*   *   *

The following is a case study written as a short story about one of the countless people who have been helped by this remedy: A Seattle woman takes a weekend trip to house sit on Mercer Island and slows down a yeast infection by devising a novel use for breakfast yogurt.

"Getaway"

After weeks of secret planning and relentless arm-twisting at work, she was on her way to six days housesitting a mansion boasting an indoor pool, Jacuzzi, sauna, three fireplaces, a kitchen larger than the average one-bedroom apartment, movie room, fitness room, and five bathrooms--one with a bar and a small waterfall--on grounds fronting Lake Washington. She left West Seattle just after eleven in the morning, blowing east on a warm October breeze, reveling in the rare sunny day, driving too fast and feeling cocky with freedom. The windows of her white Honda were all the way down, the radio was turned all the way up, and Eric Clapton and Creme were taking her down to the *Crossroads* on her favorite classic rock station, KZOK. All around, trees were shyly migrating from late-summer green through ladybug red to school-bus yellow. Her spirits were light as papier mache, *but no matter how far back she squeezed it, the memory of what happened would not leave her alone, turning up at all the wrong times like a shadow casting itself at will, not needing her permission to exist.*
She took I-5 north to 90 east and crossed the Lacey V. Murrow

Floating Bridge, which empties onto the northern shore of Mercer Island, a tony little enclave for Seattle's upper middle class and higher. Five miles long and two and a quarter miles at its widest point in the north, its shape is reminiscent of Italy, except that it looks less like a boot and more like the shoe where the old woman in the fairy tale lived. It is largely populated by gated estates, variously configured mansions set back from the street, customized luxury homes, and a small number of newly-built condos. Since the late 70's a few more modest areas have crept in, but even before the influx of California immigrants started driving up real estate prices, Mercer Island had some of the most costly homes in the Seattle area.

She took the second exit on the island at 77th Avenue Southeast and slowed down, scanning for a shopping center. She was still close to I-90, which loped across the northern shore like an asphalt necklace, and wasn't sure what she would find further south in the way of shopping possibilities. After just a few blocks she spotted a QFC supermarket located in a larger shopping center and pulled into the parking lot. As she stepped from the car, a slight wind swept over her carrying the strong cool odors of pine and damp soil. When she breathed deeper she could smell the fresh water of Lake Washington a few blocks away.

As she roamed the grocery aisles, letting her eyes slide over the merchandise, she thought about the next five days of stolen liberty. She would spend the entire time in pure solitude, reading, soaking in the Jacuzzi, staring at a fire or the lake, watching movies, having no contact with the outside world. *No contact with him.* Boo's parents would be gone all month so the phone wasn't in service. She remembered his request that she keep her cell phone turned on and opened her shoulder bag to double check, making sure the power was *off.*

She was very good at doing nothing, could sit quietly for hours by herself staring out a window--or at a wall--strolling the familiar, but always novel, corridors of her mind. She longed for days when she didn't have to leave her apartment--when she had done all the food shopping, mailed the bills, picked up the dry cleaning, filled the prescription, and returned the videos, when there was no good reason to go out. *If she could catch him at work, he was good for picking up last minute forgotten items. But he didn't know how to shop--too impulsive, wouldn't follow the list.* Stop! She shook her head, trying to dispel these treacherous thoughts, and turned into the cookie aisle, reaching immediately for ginger snaps, enticed by the promise of "real ginger and molasses" on the front of the box. Make that two boxes. She added a package of Oreos and one of Pecan Sandies. Another indulgence she permitted herself on vacations was forgetting about calorie counts.

As she waited in the check-out line she noted the contents of her basket: in addition to the cookies there were sourdough and whole wheat breads, a whole roasted chicken, deli-sliced turkey and Swiss cheese, jars of mayonnaise, mustard, blackberry jam, and honey, two cans of ripe olives, head of iceberg and one of radicchio, an onion, cucumber, and two tomatoes, bunch of bananas, bag of plums, two cans of tuna packed in water, bottle of vinaigrette dressing, half-dozen eggs, turkey bacon, stick of salted butter, assorted flavors of Dannon yogurt-- the kind with the fruit on the bottom, 1% milk, ginger ale, raisin bran, a half-gallon of Dreyer's Homemade Chocolate Chip ice cream, three bottles of Pouilly Fuisse, fire starter logs, and Tampax. It was more than she could use in six days, but having too much was the whole point.

The bag of plums caught her attention for a second time and she reached for them, thinking, *I hate plums! He eats plums.* She grabbed the suddenly despicable fruit and plunked it down in the rack holding the last copy of an "Enquirer." The cover pictured an 85-year-old woman holding the monkey boy she had supposedly birthed. The bright-eyed cashier pretended not to notice and asked, "How're you doing this afternoon?" as she placed her groceries on the moving conveyor belt.

Three hours later she was nude, up to her elbows in hot churning water, brushing cookie crumbs from her chin, and several chapters into her first read, *Imzadi.* Elliot Bay Book Company was having a sale on *Star Trek--Next Generation* paperbacks, and the last time she was downtown she'd bought three just for this occasion. This book explored the origins of the sexual tension between Counselor Troy and Commander Riker so evident on the television series. Like a good meal that had to be eaten slowly to be savored and enjoyed, she didn't want to read too fast. She was bent on pure escapism for the coming days, perhaps because her job exposed her to so much stress and potential confrontation. *It was supposed to be a well deserved getaway for two.*

She languished in the Jacuzzi for hours, reading and eating

ginger snaps. When she finally emerged, the skin on the bottom of both feet was prune puckered and her body temperature felt like 110 degrees. She dried off and pulled on a downy sweat suit smelling nicely of detergent; it was pale blue, soft and warm against her damp skin. Her lower abdomen was cramped, and she knew she'd get her period in the next twenty-four hours. She took two Motrin and went through the motions of unpacking the rest of her jumbled suitcase. *After all that meticulous planning she'd packed in angry haste, forgetting half her clothes and toiletries.*

While looking in a walk-in closet for a place to stow her suitcase, she found an old style record player and a waist high stack of long playing vinyl records, mostly the blues. *Perfect.* But first she wanted a fire. She rubbed her hands together happily when she found plenty of cut timber--good, dry cedar logs--in a cherry-wood bunker tucked in a corner to the right of the fireplace. It still took longer than she expected to start a fire, even with the help of the starter logs. Was the flue supposed to be open? They always made this s--- look so easy in movies.

When the flames were two feet high and the fire blazing hot, she dragged out the record player and set it up on an immense cherry-wood coffee table. She placed a tall stack on the turntable--Muddy Waters, Bobby Blue Bland, B.B. King, and John Lee Hooker. Muddy opened with... *"A summer day, sweet summer's day. Gone and left meeeee, girl said she's gone to stay. Well, she's goooooone, but I don't worrorrry, 'cause I'm siiitting on tooop of the world."* The music floated out from the small speakers and hung in the air like early morning mist, the lyrics reminding her why she was there alone. *There it was again, swelling her heart.* With difficulty she moved her thoughts away from the subject, refusing to let it ruin her holiday. All she knew for certain was lying never worked, no matter how bad the bloody truth.

Cavernous windows, and the placement of a fireplace in the front and center of the great room, made it possible to gaze simultaneously at the fire, the lake, and the sky. She was settled on a bank of pillows, gazing across the water where intermittent lights of cars moved along Seward Park Avenue, and a plane climbed silently into the night over Boeing Field.

What concerned her now was a very personal itch that was worsening rapidly, making her increasingly uncomfortable. She was forced to keep her legs parted or it was unbearable. Between the oncoming period and the hot Jacuzzi water, she had the beginning of a nasty yeast infection. She had seen her doctor and was using an over-the-counter medication; *that was one of the items she forgot to pack.* But she was cocooned now, didn't want to go out.

A half hour later she stood at the open refrigerator door pondering what to nosh next. Her gaze fell on the four containers of Dannon yogurt on the top shelf. She selected blueberry and shut the refrigerator door while an idea formed. Breakfast yogurt is essentially bacteria culture with milk solids and fruit, the same bacteria that inhabits the human intestinal tract and keeps it healthy. Maybe, she thought, yogurt would work on her itching--which was no more than a pH imbalance--the way it worked in the intestines. Leaving the blueberry fruit unstirred on the bottom, she used the plain yogurt as a topical ointment.

The yogurt didn't work to her complete satisfaction--it was messy, sticky, and sometimes stung her sensitive vaginal tissue--but it gave her enough relief so she didn't have to go out. She continued to spend several hours each day in the Jacuzzi without discomfort. The results encouraged her to investigate further. She remembered seeing Acidophilus sold in health foods stores and knew it was comparable to the live lactobacillus cultures found in yogurt. On her way home Monday afternoon she stopped at Puget Consumers Coop, on California Avenue, and bought a large bottle of Acidophilus softgels.

At home there was a single red rose in a newly-purchased crystal vase sitting beside her computer. She picked up the rose and smelled its sweet fragrance, replacing it without reading the note propped against the vase. She went into the small bathroom and fished around in the cabinet drawers until she found a small pair of nail scissors. She washed her hands and between her legs, snipped the top off two softgels, and was delighted and relieved when the Acidophilus worked almost upon contact. The relief was so heartfelt she groaned in pleasure. Turning her face to the ceiling she let out a sigh. What a relief. She didn't know how bad it felt until it stopped.

She washed her hands again and retraced her steps to the living room, returning to the rose in the vase. She stared at the folded note for a while before picking it up lightly between index and middle fingers and walking with it to the oversized sofa to sit down. *What could he possibly say that would change anything?*

She opened the note, read it quickly, and dropped it onto the sofa beside her. *He was good, she'd give him that.* Of all the words he could have said, he'd picked the right ones. They hadn't been together long enough for her to know whether the note was truth or tactic. Time would decide that, she need only wait. For now, there wasn't anything she would rather have him say and mean, not even "I love you," than what he'd written, *"I promise, it won't happen again."*

CHAPTER 9

LECITHIN

• **Relieve Angina Pain And Help Prevent Heart Attacks**

• **Clean Out Blocked Arteries And Heart Valves Without Surgery**

• **Help Prevent Bloodclot Stroke**

• **Lower Cholesterol**

• **Clear Up Lung And Sinus Congestion**

• **Protect Your Liver From Fatty Deposits**

• **Help Avoid Gallstones**

• **Guard Against The Harmful Effects Of Eating Red Meat And Other Foods Containing Saturated Fats**

• **Loosen Stiff Arthritic Joints And End Gout**
    Healing Osteoarthritis
    Fighting Rheumatoid Arthritis

Lecithin is a natural food substance extracted from soybean oil.

Its primary function in the body is to create and sustain an environment where oil and water can mix, given their known properties to repel each other. Oils and fats are essential for good health, yet they must function in your watery internal environment. Lecithin makes this possible by acting as your body's emulsifier. Each Lecithin molecule binds with a fat molecule and prevents it from joining with other fat molecules by holding it in suspension while it travels through your body. Without sufficient Lecithin in your system, oils, fats, and other organic compounds can clump together, solidify, and clog up your arteries, joints, lungs, liver, and other vital areas.

Lecithin can prevent cholesterol molecules from settling on the walls of your arteries, building up plaque, forming blood clots, and shutting off the blood and oxygen supply to your heart and brain--a primary cause of many conditions including angina, heart attack, and stroke. Doctors estimate that of the six hundred thousand Americans who suffer strokes each year, eighty percent are caused by a clot obstructing bloodflow.

Lecithin can also lower cholesterol, and dissolve gallstones-- which are essentially hardened balls of cholesterol. According to a recent issue of *TIME* Magazine, patients on cholesterol-lowering and other heart medications fail to fill their prescriptions forty percent of the time. After five years half stop taking the drugs altogether, blaming unpleasant side-effects as a primary reason.

In your lungs and sinus, Lecithin can clear up mucous, relieving pressure and making it easier to breathe. It can also relieve the pain and swelling of gout, and break down the protein and mineral deposits found in arthritic joints, increasing your mobility. Lecithin can help keep fatty deposits from forming in your liver, and help you avoid many of the harmful effects of eating red meat and other foods containing saturated fats.

Taken as directed, Lecithin can prevent the formation of these dangerous deposits *any place in your body*. It can also clean them out *after* they have accumulated, working surprisingly fast to cleanse the body of blockages, clots, mucous, and obstructions that stiffen joints. Lecithin can produce extraordinary benefits in your cardiovascular system. The best news is that it is known to be safe and without side effects--it has been used in our food supply over half a century--because your body can safely excrete any excess. Check your kitchen shelves and refrigerator, and you will find many products that contain it, such as dry mixes, packaged foods, ice cream, candy bars, frozen dinners, and bread products.

Recommended Strength[17]

1200 mg--from soybeans *only*. (Should contain a minimum 730 mg phosphatides, 730/1200), or approximately sixty-one percent phosphatides.[18])

Recommended Form

Softgels; granules may also be used.[19]

Taken How

Softgels: with eight ounces of juice or other liquids as directed.

Granules: sprinkled over cereal or mixed in blender drinks as directed.

Side Effects

None observed when taken as directed.

---

17 For Lecithin softgels the author has had the best results with Country Life®, Hauppauge, NY 11788, (800) 645-5768, Puritan's Pride®, Oakdale, NY 11769, (800) 645-1030, Solary®, Park City, UT 84068, and Solgar®, Leonia, NJ 07605, (800) 645-2246. Puritan's Pride is available by mail order only. The other brands can be purchased at most health foods stores and sometimes in the health foods section of supermarkets.

18 The value of a Lecithin product is determined by the percentage of phosphatides it contains, because they activate the fat emulsifying process in your body.

19 For Lecithin granules, the author has had the best results with Nature's Food Farm®, Los Angeles, CA 90066, available in most health foods stores, or in the health foods section of supermarkets.

Notes√√

√ Lecithin softgels are somewhat large but very smooth, and they go down easily with a swallow of liquid when taken one at a time.

√ Although softgels are the recommended form, you may also use Lecithin granules, which are less expensive and more potent, though not as convenient. A one pound bag is usually priced less than $5. You can use granules to augment your daily intake, or as a substitute for one or more of the daily doses of softgels. (One tablespoon equals 7500 mg with a phosphatide content of ninety-five percent; six softgels equal 7200 mg with a minimum phosphatide content of sixty-one percent.) Granules can be sprinkled over or mixed in a variety of foods, but may change their consistency. They are best used in cereals or mixed in blender drinks, because they do not dissolve easily in liquids. Lecithin granules used in cooking cannot be counted toward your daily intake for purposes of the remedy.

√ It is a common belief that eggs are not healthy due to their high levels of cholesterol. But, in addition to cholesterol, the yolk also contains enough Lecithin to counteract the ill effects of most of that cholesterol, provided it is not cooked "well done." Prepare your eggs soft boiled, sunny side, over easy, or even over medium, to retain the beneficial effects of the natural Lecithin.

•Relieve Angina Pain And Help Prevent Heart Attacks

•Clean Out Blocked Arteries And Heart Valves Without Surgery

•Help Prevent Bloodclot Stroke

•Lower Cholesterol

1. Take 7200 mg (6 softgels) of Lecithin four times daily, i.e., 8:00 am, noon, 4:00 pm, 8:00 pm, and continue for four weeks. (If you are treating angina pain, continue at this level until the painful episodes have stopped for at least two weeks.)

2. Reduce to 7200 mg (6 softgels) three times daily, morning, afternoon, and evening, and continue for twelve weeks.

3. Reduce to 6000 mg (5 softgels) three times daily, morning, afternoon, and evening, and continue for four weeks.

4. Reduce to 6000 mg (5 softgels) twice daily, morning and evening, and continue as a maintenance dose to help keep your cardiovascular system unblocked.

Remedy At A Glance (Lecithin)

	8:00 am	Noon	4:00 pm	8:00 pm
Daily For Four Weeks To Relieve Symptoms:	7200 mg	7200 mg	7200 mg	7200 mg

	Morning	Afternoon	Evening	
Daily For Twelve Weeks To Relieve Symptoms:	7200 mg	7200 mg	7200 mg	
Daily For Four Weeks To Relieve Symptoms:	6000 mg	6000 mg	6000 mg	
Daily As A Maintenance Dose:	6000 mg		6000 mg	

Notes√√

√ If you have any of the cardiovascular conditions mentioned, *you should be under the care of a physician.* Do not rely solely on nutritional supplements to treat these dangerous disorders.

√ To help heal a cardiovascular condition, it is recommended that you also take **Beta Carotene** and **Vitamin E Complex**. Beta Carotene accelerates healing anywhere in the body, and Vitamin E Complex specifically supports healing in the heart and cardiovascular system.

Beta Carotene: Use in 25,000 IU softgels only. Take it once a day with your largest meal as directed, regardless of the amount you are taking.

1. Take 250,000 IU (10 softgels) daily, and continue for five days.

2. Reduce to 200,000 IU (8 softgels) daily, and continue for one week.

3. Reduce to 175,000 IU (7 softgels) daily, and continue for two weeks.

154

4. Reduce to 150,000 IU (6 softgels) daily, and continue for two weeks.

5. Reduce to 125,000 IU (5 softgels) daily, and continue for two weeks.

6. Reduce to 100,000 IU (4 softgels) daily, and continue for four weeks.

7. Continue to take 75,000 IU (3 softgels) daily, as a maintenance dose to help keep your cardiovascular system healthy.

Remedy At A Glance (Beta Carotene)

	Once A Day With Largest Meal
Daily For Five Days To Relieve Symptoms:	250,000 IU
Daily For One Week To Relieve Symptoms:	200,000 IU
Daily For Two Weeks To Relieve Symptoms:	175,000 IU
Daily For Two Weeks To Relieve Symptoms:	150,000 IU
Daily For Two Weeks To Relieve Symptoms:	125,000 IU
Daily For Four Weeks To Relieve Symptoms:	100,000 IU
Daily As A Maintenance Dose:	75,000 IU

See Chapter 5 for more on Beta Carotene and how to use it as a remedy to shorten healing time by more than half, and *drastically* reduce wound tenderness and scarring.

Vitamin E Complex: Use in 400 IU, softgels only, *mixed* tocopherols only.[20] Take it once a day with food as directed, regardless of the amount you are taking.

1. Take 1200 IU daily, and continue for four weeks.

2. Reduce to 800 IU daily, and continue as a maintenance dose to support good health in your cardiovascular system.

Remedy At A Glance (Vitamin E Complex)

	Once A Day
Daily For Four Weeks To Strengthen Heart:	1200 IU
Daily As A Maintenance Dose:	800 IU

See Volume II of this series for more on Vitamin E Complex and how to use it to support a healthy cardiovascular system.

•Clear Up Lung And Sinus Congestion

1. Take 6000 mg (5 softgels) of Lecithin three times daily, morning, afternoon, and evening, and continue as long as you have any sinus discomfort or congestion in your lungs.

2. Reduce to 6000 mg (5 softgels) twice daily, morning and

---

20 For Vitamin E Complex the author has had the best results with Country Life®, Hauppauge, NY 11788, (800) 645-5768, Puritan's Pride®, Oakdale, NY 11769, (800) 645-1030, Solgar®, Leonia, NJ 07605, (800) 645-2246, and Twinlab®, Ronkonkoma, NY 11779, (800) 645-5626. Puritan's Pride is available by mail order only. The other brands can be purchased at most health foods stores and sometimes in the health foods section of supermarkets.

evening, and continue for one week.

3. At this point you may discontinue Lecithin, or continue to take 4800 mg (4 softgels) twice daily, morning and evening, as a maintenance dose to help keep your lungs and sinus clear of congestion.

Remedy At A Glance (Lecithin)

	Morning	Afternoon	Evening
Daily To Relieve Congestion:	6000 mg	6000 mg	6000 mg
Daily For One Week After You Are Better:	6000 mg		6000 mg
Daily As A Maintenance Dose: (Optional)	4800 mg		4800 mg

•Protect Your Liver From Fatty Deposits

•Help Avoid Gallstones

•Guard Against The Harmful Effects Of Eating Red Meat And Other Foods Containing Saturated Fats

1. Take 6000 mg (5 softgels) of Lecithin twice daily, morning and evening, and continue as a maintenance dose to protect yourself from these conditions.

2. As an extra precaution, take 2400 mg (2 softgels) per serving, directly after you eat foods containing saturated fats, such as red meat, butter, fried foods, pork products, etc. This is in addition to your daily maintenance dose.

Remedy At A Glance (Lecithin)

	Morning	Evening
Daily As A Maintenance Dose:	6000 mg	6000 mg

	Directly After You Eat
Additional Per Serving Of Food With Saturated Fats:	2400 mg

•Loosen Stiff Arthritic Joints And End Gout

1. Take 7200 mg (6 softgels) of Lecithin four times daily, i.e., 8:00 am, noon, 4:00 pm, 8:00 pm, and continue for four weeks.

2. Reduce to 7200 mg (6 softgels) three times daily, morning, afternoon, and evening, and continue as long as you have any symptoms.

3. Reduce to 7200 mg (6 softgels) twice daily, morning and evening, and continue as a maintenance dose to help keep your joints healthy and free-moving, and to help prevent gout.

Remedy At A Glance (Lecithin)

	8:00 am	Noon	4:00 pm	8:00 pm
Daily For Four Weeks To Relieve Symptoms:	7200 mg	7200 mg	7200 mg	7200 mg

	Morning	Afternoon	Evening
Daily To Relieve Symptoms:	7200 mg	7200 mg	7200 mg

	Morning		Evening
Daily As A Maintenance Dose:	7200 mg		7200 mg

Healing Osteoarthritis

If you are treating osteoarthritis, it is recommended that you also take **Glucosamine Sulfate** and **Chondroitin Sulfate**. These two supplements can heal and promote good health in joints ravaged by this disorder. Glucosamine Sulfate is the actual substance your body needs to repair joints; Chondroitin Sulfate instructs your body to make its own Glucosamine. Taken in combination, they give you the best chance for fast healing. These are some of the highest priced supplements on the market, but their benefits are completely worth the cost.

Glucosamine Sulfate and Chondroitin Sulfate Taken Together In Combination: Use Glucosamine Sulfate in 1000 mg, capsule form only; use Chondroitin Sulfate in 500 mg, capsule form only.[21] Take them with juice or other liquids as directed.

1. Take 4000 mg (4 capsules) of Glucosamine Sulfate, and 2000 mg (4 capsules) of Chondroitin Sulfate (a **"double dose"**) each morning, and continue until your symptoms are gone.

2. Reduce to 2000 mg (2 capsules) of Glucosamine Sulfate, and 1000 mg (2 capsules) of Chondroitin Sulfate (a **"single dose"**) each morning, and continue as a maintenance dose to help keep your joints healthy.

3. Because Sulfates work better when taken with Vitamin C, it is recommended that you take 2000 mg of Vitamin C Complex with each double dose, and 1000 mg with each single dose.

Remedy At A Glance (Glucosamine Sulfate And Chondroitin Sulfate)

	Each Morning	
Daily To Relieve Symptoms:	Double Dose	(Plus 2000 mg Vitamin C Complex)
Daily As A Maintenance Dose:	Single Dose	(Plus 1000 mg Vitamin C Complex)

---

21 The author has had the best results with Puritan's Pride® Glucosamine Sulfate and Chondroitin Sulfate, Oakdale, NY 11769, available by mail order only at (800) 645-1030.

See Volume II of this series for more on these Sulfates and how to use them to heal and prevent osteoarthritis.

See Chapter 3 and Chapter 7 for more on Vitamin C Complex, and how to us it in combination with other supplements to heal numerous conditions.

Fighting Rheumatoid Arthritis

If you are treating rheumatoid arthritis, a serious auto-immune disorder, it is recommended that you also take five to six additional food supplements: **Beta Carotene, L-Cysteine And Vitamin C Complex, Bee Pollen, Vitamin B12,** and sometimes **Iron.** Beta Carotene helps relieve inflammation, heal damage to bone and soft tissue, and eliminate pain, swelling, and tenderness. L-Cysteine and Vitamin C Complex, taken together, accelerate detoxification and assist Lecithin in excreting the organic "debris" removed from the joints. Bee Pollen strengthens and helps promote good health in the immune system, *without triggering an auto immune response*. Vitamin B12 helps alleviate the debilitating fatigue associated with this disorder. Iron helps eliminate the anemia experienced by many who have it. (If you know your red blood cell count is normal you do not need to take Iron.)

For this remedy to work it is crucial that you keep your system flooded with the supplements. You can feel worse after missing even one day of dosages.

Beta Carotene: Use in 25,000 IU softgels only. Take it once a day with your largest meal as directed, regardless of the amount you are taking.

1. Take 250,000 IU (10 softgels) daily, for the first two days of each week, i.e., Sunday and Monday.

2. Reduce to 200,000 IU (8 softgels) daily, for the next three days, i.e., Tuesday, Wednesday, and Thursday.

3. Reduce to 150,000 IU (6 softgels) daily, for the last two

days, i.e., Friday and Saturday.

4. Continue at this level until your symptoms are gone.

5. Reduce to 100,000 IU (4 softgels) daily, and continue as a maintenance dose to help maintain good health in your joints.

Remedy At A Glance (Beta Carotene)

Once A Day With Largest Meal

	Days 1-2	Days 3-5	Days 6-7
Daily To Relieve Symptoms:	250,000 IU	200,000 IU	150,000 IU
Daily As A Maintenance Dose:		100,000 IU	

See Chapter 5 for more on Beta Carotene and how to use it as a remedy to shorten healing time by more than half, and *drastically* reduce wound tenderness and scarring.

L-Cysteine And Vitamin C Complex Taken Together In Combination: Use 500 mg tablets or capsules of L-Cysteine; use 1000 mg tablets or capsules of Vitamin C Complex. They should be taken together--at the same time--with juice or other liquids as directed. The amount of Vitamin C Complex should always equal twice that of L-Cysteine. You may use Vitamin C alone, without the other trace elements, if you cannot find Vitamin C Complex.

1. Take 500 mg of L-Cysteine and 1000 mg of Vitamin C Complex (a "single dose"), four times daily, i.e., 8:00 am, noon, 4:00 pm, 8:00 pm, and continue for four weeks.

2. Reduce to a single dose three times daily, morning, afternoon, and evening, and continue until your symptoms are gone.

3. Reduce to a single dose twice daily, morning and evening, and continue as a maintenance dose to help maintain good health in your joints.

161

Remedy At A Glance (L-Cysteine And Vitamin C Complex)

	8:00 am	Noon	4:00 pm	8:00 pm
Daily For Four Weeks To Relieve Symptoms:	Single Dose	Single Dose	Single Dose	Single Dose
	Morning	Afternoon	Evening	
Daily To Relieve Symptoms:	Single Dose	Single Dose	Single Dose	
Daily As A Maintenance Dose :	Single Dose		Single Dose	

See Chapter 3 for more on L-Cysteine and Vitamin C Complex and how to use this powerful combination as a remedy for asthma and other respiratory disorders, to guard against cigarette smoker's damage, to prevent hangovers, and to protect against liver/age spots, and environmental toxins.

Bee Pollen: Use 1000 mg pressed pellet tablets. Take it with juice or other liquids as directed.

1. Take 1000 mg four times daily, i.e., 8:00 am, noon, 4:00 pm, 8:00 pm, and continue for four weeks.

2. Reduce to 1000 mg three times daily, morning, afternoon, and evening, and continue until your symptoms are gone.

3. Reduce to 1000 mg twice daily, morning and evening, and continue as a maintenance dose to strengthen your immune system and improve resistance.

Remedy At A Glance (Bee Pollen)

	8:00 am	Noon	4:00 pm	8:00 pm
Daily For Four Weeks To Relieve Symptoms:	1000 mg	1000 mg	1000 mg	1000 mg
	Morning	Afternoon	Evening	
Daily To Relieve Symptoms:	1000 mg	1000 mg	1000 mg	
Daily As A Maintenance Dose:	1000 mg		1000 mg	

See Chapter 7 for more on Bee Pollen and how to use it with Vitamin C Complex to heal and prevent colds, improve resistance, and fight allergies, hay fever, and sinus problems--including headaches.

Vitamin B12: Use in 1000 mcg tablets, capsules, or sublingual form. Take it with eight ounces of juice or other liquids as directed. (Sublingual is dissolved under the tongue and requires no liquids.)

1. Take 2000 mcg in the morning, and 2000 mcg in the early afternoon, and continue until your symptoms are gone.

2. Reduce to 2000 mcg in the morning, 1000 mcg in the early afternoon, and continue as a maintenance dose to help fight fatigue.

Remedy At A Glance (Vitamin B12)

	Morning	Early Afternoon
Daily To Relieve Fatigue:	2000 mcg	2000 mcg
Daily A Maintenance Dose:	2000 mcg	1000 mcg

See Chapter 11 for more on Vitamin B12 and how to use it to help prevent fatigue and stop tingling extremities.

If you take Vitamin B12 for more than a few days at a time, it is recommended that you also take **Vitamin B Complex** to avoid

163

depleting other elements of the B Complex and causing a different deficiency than the one you are treating. You do not have to take B Complex and B12 together--at the same time. Be aware that B Complex can turn urine a darker yellow due to the concentration of nutrients present in B vitamins; and this is not cause for alarm.

Vitamin B Complex: Use B Complex 100, tablets or capsules.[22] (Some B vitamins included in the 100 complex are measured in milligrams, others in micrograms, but all will be contained in one tablet or capsule.) Vitamin B Complex is available in higher strength formulas, up to B Complex 150, and you may use a higher strength formula if you wish. Take it with food, because it can be hard to digest.

1. Take one tablet or capsule once a day, and continue as a maintenance dose as long as you take Vitamin B12.

Remedy At A Glance (Vitamin B Complex)

Daily As A Maintenance Dose While Taking B12:	Once A Day With Food
	B Complex 100 (or higher)

See Volume II of this series for more on Vitamin B Complex and how to use it as a remedy for certain kinds of nervousness, including muscle tics and trembling in your extremities.

Iron: Use 15 mg tablets from ferrous gluconate, which is generally easier to digest than ferrous sulfate.[23] Take it once a day with food. It can take approximately four weeks for your body to use the Iron to make enough new blood cells to raise your red blood cell count.

---

22 For Vitamin B Complex, the author has had the best results with Country Life®, Hauppauge, NY 11788, (800) 645-5768; Puritan's Pride®, Oakdale, NY 11769, (800) 645-1030; and Solgar®, Leonia, NJ 07605, (800) 645-2246. Puritan's Pride is available by mail order only. The other brands can be purchased at most health foods stores and sometimes in the health foods section of supermarkets.

23 There are too many quality brands of Iron available to mention here. Try to buy one that does not use fillers and a lot of "other ingredients."

1. Take 15 mg daily, and continue as long as your red blood cell count is below normal: 12 to 14 for women, and 14 to 16 for men.

2. Reduce to 15 mg every other day, and continue as a maintenance dose to avoid anemia.

3. Before you take an Iron supplement, be sure you do not have a genetic condition called hemochromatosis, which causes you to absorb too much Iron from food (seventy-five percent instead of the average ten to fifteen percent). The excess Iron can actually start to rust inside your body and can be very toxic.

Remedy At A Glance (Iron)

	Once A Day With Food
Daily To Raise Red Blood Cell Count:	15 mg
Every Other Day As A Maintenance Dose:	15 mg

See Volume II of this series for more on Iron and how to use it to treat anemia and fatigue.

If you experience constipation while taking Iron, see Chapter 12 for information on Magnesium Oxide and how to use it to prevent the condition.

*   *   *

The following is a case study written as a short story about one of the countless people who have been helped by this remedy: A San Diego nursing student facing the possibility of life in a wheelchair uses Lecithin and other nutritional supplements to help heal rheumatoid arthritis when drug treatments stop working and her disease worsens.

"Steely Courageous"

Susan's body hammered at her senses, the pain shrieking hotly into her joints with a fury that left her weak and breathless. She leaned against the porcelain sink for support, wanting to wash her hands but dreading the suffering that twisting the faucets would unleash in her shoulders and fingers. Nausea bubbled in her stomach, one side effect of the drugs she was taking to treat rheumatoid arthritis. The door to the locker room swooshed open and two interns walked in, trailing an antiseptic aroma and discussing an autopsy they had just witnessed. Like Susan, they were nursing students at Pacific West College, working two days a week in the wards at St. Christopher's Medical Center. She turned on the faucet and hurriedly washed her hands. Using the wall-mounted soap dispenser made her shoulders scream in protest, and she had to concentrate on her breathing to remain quiet.

"Hey Sue, how are you doing?" Indira asked, coming to stand beside her classmate while she checked her make-up in the mirror. She extracted a comb from her shoulder bag and pulled it through her waist-length black hair. A faded, worn denim jacket covered the top of her tan and gold sari.

Having been raised to keep her complaints to herself, Susan smiled brightly, saying, "Never been better. How about you?"

"Don't ask. You were smart not to attend the chop job. I fear it has seriously disturbed my stomach," Indira said, with the rhythm of Bombay dancing in her words.

"Ooh, I'm so sorry you don't feel well. I have mints, would they help?" Susan asked.

"No, don't trouble yourself. I am going to the cafeteria for a cup of tea and some soup after I change." Indira held a plastic, dry-cleaning bag in the crook of two fingers. In it were the white slacks, white shirt, and blue vest nursing students wore. "I was afraid to eat beforehand," she said. "Didn't know if it would stay put."

After Indira headed off to find her locker, Susan started for the door twenty-five feet away. She glanced around, saw no one, and immediately relaxed her guard, submitting to the pain wailing in her ankles and knees with each step. With her face grimaced in distress, she walked on the outer sides of her feet, mincing along this way because her ankles could no longer make a complete rotation. Her arms were held stiffly by her sides to avoid shoulder movement. When she reached the door she took a deep breath, straightened up, and joined the flow in the busy corridor, her gait nearly normal now if you didn't look too close.

She went directly to a water fountain, popped two Tylenol in her mouth and bent to drink, holding her long, blond hair away from the spout, reminding herself she had now taken eight and it was only 2:30 p.m. The pain killers only dulled the agony in her joints which never stopped.

"So here you are. I've been looking all over." Nurse Mabel Watson stood with a scowl on her black face, strong hands resting on stout hips, her church-woman's bosom heaving from the fast walk, her hair a halo of red frizzy curls.

"You're supposed to be assisting Dr. Medley with a pelvic exam in 402. Not pulling your little disappearing act again," she said.

Susan was startled and swallowed the wrong way, causing a spasm of coughing. Trying to be helpful, Nurse Watson pounded her back hard enough to break a rib. Susan turned around, backing away from her, holding up a hand to indicate she was alright, though she still coughed. She composed herself and smiling weakly, offered, "Mr. Reynolds was waiting in the hallway over an hour for someone to take him down to X-ray. I mean, this poor man. Said it hurt his back sitting up in the wheelchair, you know? So I'm all, like, I'm sure it would be okay if ... "

Nurse Watson cut her off. "You are here to follow my orders. Suppose an emergency had occurred when I needed you and couldn't find you? Did you ever think of that?"

"I'm sorry," Susan said, trying to imagine an emergency where the presence of a first-year nursing student would make a difference.

"It is important I know where all my interns are at all times," Nurse Watson growled.

Talking too loud, she continued, "And what about your hair? Just because we're in southern California doesn't mean we're going to adopt lazy beach attitudes. Not while I'm Nurse Supervisor. You know long hair is supposed to be in a bun or braided. Now get along. Doctor is waiting for you."

Nurse Watson's charcoal complexion shone with a momentary vitality that faded as soon as her words escaped. She watched Susan nod before turning to depart, and shook her head, wondering why the young woman wasn't the star pupil she had been at the start.

"And when you're through with the pelvic, clean the bedpans on ward A before you leave," she called out, before turning to stride purposefully in the other direction.

Susan could have pointed out that Indira's hair was several inches longer that hers, or that one of the male students wore his woolly tresses Rastafarian style, while two other men had manes well past their shoulders, and no one was asking them for buns and braids--but she didn't. She also didn't tell Nurse Watson the real reason, that she *couldn't*. Her fiancé, Jess, had tried a couple of mornings--proudly brushing, looping, and pinning--but it always fell out before she reached her car in the parking lot.

A few minutes past four, Susan stood in front of her locker, beginning to relax, knowing she'd made it through another hospital day without being discovered. A moment later her pager vibrated. She walked slowly to the wall phone at the end of the aisle and dialed Nurse Watson. When she hung up she began to tremble, and her blue eyes filled with water.

Indira appeared from another row of lockers. "What on earth has made you cry, Sue?" she asked, placing a brown hand gently on each shoulder of Susan's petite frame.

That small act of concern broke Susan's defenses and she began to cry in earnest. "My arthritis has gotten worse, a lot worse."

"What arthritis? I didn't know you had arthritis," Indira said, and produced a clean handkerchief to wipe away the tears that fell on Susan's cheeks.

"Watson wants me down in ER to draw blood. I don't think I can, you know, hold on to the needles anymore. The last time ... I-I almost .... I know I should tell her, I can't risk endangering a patient. But if I tell her the truth ... she will, like, totally get rid of me. She already hates me."

"No one hates you, little one. But first things first. I will accompany you to the emergency room and do whatever you cannot. It will be our secret. Now calm yourself, please."

*   *   *

When Susan got home she went right to the medicine cabinet

168

for Tylenol and took two. From there she went to the kitchen, where a note from Jess sat on a Formica counter top. He'd gone to Vons for groceries and would be right back. She found a bottle of Blanc de Blanc chilling in the refrigerator. Thankfully, Jess had already popped the cork, so she had only a little trouble dislodging it--using the pads of her thumbs while sitting in a chair and holding the bottle between her legs-- and pouring herself a badly-needed glass.

She turned on the radio and using the backs of two fingers spun the dial, stopping at an easy listening station out of Los Angeles, playing Sade's, "Never As Good As The First Time." She unlocked the sliding glass door and took her wine outside to the small, second-floor terrace. A swelling Pacific Ocean was visible two blocks away, past the strip mall on Ocean Walk. The tide was high, and the blue-green surf foamed against the beach leaving seaweed, driftwood, and an occasional soda can at the water's edge. The air was misty and smelled of salt as it breezed through palm trees, making dried fronds crackle like a bonfire. A bank of pinkish grey clouds migrated slowly from the west.

Susan sat in a white, plastic deck chair, carefully kicked off her shoes and propped her feet on the iron railing to watch the sun go down. What a relief to get the weight off her ankles. She breathed deeply, letting the marine air wash her lungs and scrub the sour smell of filled bed pans from her nostrils. Sitting there alone, sipping her wine, watching the sky darken under somber clouds, she reluctantly gave in to the knowledge she'd been fighting for a long time. And the truth revealed itself to her without shame, as though it had been waiting for this moment to slip into her awareness.

Memories began to overtake her like the tide consuming the shoreline: The one week camping trip to the mountains of central Mexico with friends six years ago, a twenty-first birthday present from her parents; getting sick with a gastrointestinal virus the last day--the locals laughingly calling it Montezuma's revenge; then back home with the first symptoms, swollen joints, skin rashes, fever, that went away after a few weeks only to return harshly six months later; then a biopsy of a finger joint showing she had rheumatoid arthritis--she'd always thought it was a disease you were born with, had no idea you could *catch* it, like the flu; then the slow, cruel deterioration of her body.

Susan had been on the swim team in high school, played soccer, and was a long distance runner on the All-City track team.

Summers, she earned money for school clothes by lifeguarding at local beaches. But the disease robbed her of all that. Seemed like one moment she was running beside the ocean, sweet salt air rushing into her lungs, making her smile with the pleasure of feeling her strong body responding, and the next moment she had difficulty crossing a room.

With Indira's help she made it through today. No one thought it odd that Watson had sent two interns instead of one. But she could not depend on Indira or anyone else to cover for her ever again. She would have to quit nursing school, return to San Diego. She and Jess could probably stay with her parents in Chula Vista while they looked for another apartment. After that, she didn't know.

*   *   *

TWO MONTHS LATER

I parked my blue Escort under the elm tree in front of Marie's house in Clairmont, a bedroom community built into the west-facing hills above Mission Bay. It was 9:30, New Year's Day 1995, and the temperature was already eighty-five degrees at the shore. Though San Diego is generally a temperate seventy-two degrees, several times a year, hot winds called Santa Ana blow in from the desert, pushing the thermometer into the nineties, raising the pollen count and the hay fever index. I collected my bulging laundry basket and box of Tide from the trunk and let myself in the attached garage by entering a four-digit code into the pad. The wide door rolled up and back, exposing a two car garage with a washer and dryer on the right, behind a half wall and counter painted grey. I started my first load, sorted two more on the concrete floor, then went to the kitchen to make tea.

I was standing in front of an open cabinet searching for honey when I heard a soft voice inquire, "What are you looking for?"

I jumped and expelled a sigh. "You scared me. The honey."

Marie was standing beside me with sleep in her blue eyes, wearing a grey sweatshirt and white tights, hugging around her shoulders a pink quilt decorated with dancing teddy bears. A flowered coffee mug was in her free hand. She is a small wiry woman with a feisty will, who looks a little like Kathryn Hepburn.

"It's on the refrigerator door," she said, and went to the counter

170

to pour a second cup of coffee.

The microwave peeped and I removed the mug of chamomile tea, squeezing honey into the steamy liquid from a yellow, bear-shaped container.

"I thought no one was here," I said. "Aren't you supposed to be skiing in Colorado?"

"Mike and the kids left with my parents at six o'clock this morning. I didn't feel like going. Had a horrible deposition yesterday that ran until nine o'clock. On New Year's Eve no less. I wanted to kill opposing counsel. What a creep. Didn't want to let me enter exhibits because it was his deposition. Can you believe it?"

"I'm sure he loved you too," I said, stirring my tea.

"Well, I did my best to make his life hell, naturally," she said, and blew on her coffee.

"Naturally."

"I succeeded too. We stopped at nine because he had a migraine. I had one too, but I kept anyone else from knowing about it. Unlike that sissy," she said, and laughed loudly. Her efforts at being lighthearted told me she still had the migraine.

We sat quietly for the next few minutes, lost in our own thoughts, sipping our drinks, perched on two stools in front of a wrap-around counter that connects the kitchen to the dining area. In the garage the washer gurgled into the rinse cycle.

Marie taught me everything I know about practicing law. (Law schools teach theory mostly, and how to think like a lawyer, but the practical side is not a high priority.) She is a brilliant plaintiff's attorney who represents the "little guy" against large corporate defense firms, usually in employment discrimination actions based on race, sex, or national origin. I clerked at her firm right out of law school. We made a great team, each endowed with skills that made up for small things lacking in the other. We weren't working together now because I had my own business, but we still kept in close touch.

Out of nowhere she said, "You have to help my sister. If you don't, by this time next year she'll be in a wheelchair."

"Which one is this again?" I asked, remembering that Marie had four sisters, *and* four brothers.

"Susie, the youngest. She has rheumatoid arthritis. She's losing everything she loves, and it's killing me. I can't let that happen to her.

I practically raised her. I saw her Christmas Day. She could hardly walk. You're the only person I know who might be able to help her." Marie's voice was choked with emotion when she finished.

I returned to the garage to move wet clothes into the dryer and start a new load in the washer, thinking about what Marie said. She followed me, dragging her quilt behind like a train.

"Don't you think you can help her?" she asked, with tears in her eyes.

"Sure I can. Where's she live?" I asked, and tossed a Downy softener sheet into the dryer on top of the clothes. I had never treated rheumatoid arthritis, but I also had never seen food supplements fail to heal or improve any condition. I was excited at the prospect of working with a new subject and a new disorder.

"Near you. Ocean Beach. Why don't I set up something here for next week," Marie said, wiping her eyes, back in control. "We'll barbecue. How does that sound?"

*   *   *

Three days after my conversation with Marie, I was seated in her home office when the doorbell chimed in the front of the house. I listened to her greet her sister, saying in the distance, "Lynn's waiting in my office. I'm outside with the kids and the barbecue."

I stood, expecting Susan to appear in the doorway any second, the distance between the front door and the office being no more than thirty feet. When a full minute passed and she didn't appear, I started out of the office, assuming she'd gone into the yard with Marie. But there she was, limping along in a sort of waddle walk, face grimaced in pain, elbows bent at her sides, hands frozen in front like broken birds. When she looked up and saw me, her posture changed and she got a sheepish look, as though I'd caught her doing something she shouldn't. She tried to affect a normal stride. I walked out to meet her. We introduced ourselves and shook hands. I applied normal pressure, unwittingly hurting her enough to bring tears to her eyes. I apologized. She smiled and shook it off. It took several minutes before we were seated on a sofa in Marie's office.

The house was quiet. I could hear a clock ticking in the next room, and Elisha and Chris playing outside. The air drifting in an open window smelled of mowed grass, lighter fluid, and newly-burning charcoal. Susan wore faded jeans and white sneakers and sat with her hands hidden in the folds of a baggy green sweater. She was a little over five feet, about a hundred pounds, with a symmetrical face infused with innocence. I knew she was twenty-seven, but she looked younger. She also looked scared.

"Marie says you, like, help people get better and you're writing a book about it," she began.

I nodded. "I've helped a lot of people. Maybe I can help you too."

"You think so? Really?" she asked. "I'd try anything to get better."

"Tell me specifically how the disease effects you. I spent yesterday in the medical school library at UCSD reading about it, so I know generally what it does in the body," I said. "I need to know exactly what *your* symptoms are, and we'll start by simply treating each one."

While she talked I asked her to stand and perform a few movements so I could see the extent of her loss of mobility. She showed me she could raise both arms sideways only about forty-five degrees. She had difficulty bending her knees, and I knew from seeing her walk that her ankles were a problem. I noticed when we shook hands that several of her fingers seemed to be locked in position at odd, unnatural angles.

"If you want the remedy to work you'll have to follow some ground rules, okay?"

"Anything. I'll do anything to get better."

"You'll have to buy the brand, strength, and form that I tell you to, and follow my instructions to the letter. You can't miss even one day's dose. It will take a few weeks before you feel significant relief. After that you should get better progressively. Oh, one other thing: you'll have to take these supplements for the rest of your life, and in pretty high doses, or your symptoms will probably return."

"I have to take *drugs* the rest of my life. What's the difference? Be better off with vitamins. I wanted to ask you about the drugs, though. Don't you think I should stop taking them to, like, give the vitamins a fair chance to work?"

"That's up to you, but you don't have to. The supplements will

173

still work."

"I *want* to stop taking drugs. They don't work and I hate the side effects. Do you know I spend, like, one full day each week in the hospital getting checked and probed, just to track what they're doing inside my body. I mean, they kill my sex drive, what's up with that? They sap my energy. They totally suck."

"Which ones are you taking?" I asked.

She shifted in her seat and brought her hands out of hiding to rest on her lap. "Well, let's see. Prednisone, that's a steroid, and Methotrexate, a cancer drug--it makes me so sick. Took three kinds of gold, orally and by injection; it helped a little in the beginning, but didn't slow down the disease, after a while it stopped working." She let out a deep sigh. "And I've taken a couple of experimentals in drug trials. All I do is get worse. There's a lot of stuff they can't give me 'cause I'd like to have children someday--and there is a risk of miscarriage and infertility. I tried acupuncture. It made me feel better for a day or so; nothing long lasting so I stopped. And then there were herbs. They didn't work either and were so gross. I had to cook them for hours. I'm, like, bent over this huge pot, totally, like a witch," she said, laughing for the first time and revealing an unexpected radiance.

Marie came into the room. "Excuse me Susie, Lynn, but would you prefer to have chicken or lobster tails? Or would you like both?"

"Lobster tails!" we said at the same time.

On the long trip to the back yard, Susan stopped in the kitchen for a glass of water to wash down two Tylenol tablets.

*   *   *

Jess was waiting up for Susan when she got home. He was watching The Tonight Show, his long body stretched out on the bed on top of a beige comforter. Jay Leno was in the middle of his opening monologue, an unbroken stream of clever jokes about the O.J. Simpson trial. The audience was eating it up. Susan laid down beside Jess and went eagerly into his open arms. He used the remote to turn off the television, giving her all his attention.

"I missed you. How'd it go?" he asked in the darkness, and kissed the top of her head. His voice was soft and caring.

"Okay I guess. Lynn is really nice."

174

"Do you think she can help you?"

"Marie thinks so."

"What do you think, Susan?"

"Probably not, but I gotta try it. I'll try anything. I'm scared, Jess. I hate what the drugs are doing to my body. I like the idea that the supplements may actually heal me and not just mask my symptoms, you know?" Then a pause before saying, "I'm gonna' go for it. Maybe she can help me, you never know."

They fell asleep in each other's arms.

*   *   *

Susan immersed herself in the vitamin regimen with a singular dedication that I have rarely witnessed. I was grateful for her trust, buoyed by her enthusiasm, and amazed at her courage. She told me later that she hadn't believed the remedy would help her. But that didn't stop her from committing herself to it completely. She bought a special backpack and carried the bottles of supplements with her no matter where she went, determined not to miss a single dose. The day before she began the remedy, she decided on her own to stop using all arthritis drugs except Piroxicam, a mild prescription anti-inflammatory. I tried unsuccessfully to dissuade her, thinking it might be easier on her body if she tapered off the drugs slowly. She also continued to take Tylenol to relieve constant pain in her joints, which she measured as eight on a scale of one to ten.

Two weeks after starting the remedy, Susan reported less pain and swelling, and that she had reduced her Tylenol intake to ten daily. After thirty days, she had freer movement in joints that had previously been stiff and sometimes locked in place. She was down to six Tylenol daily, and reported that morning stiffness was reduced from two hours to thirty minutes. Marie had warned me about Susan's tendency, and her ability, to hide the truth about her disease. We met in person regularly, and she performed specific movements, so I could see for myself whether she was improving.

Susan's condition continued to get better and after six weeks it had stabilized, a nice way of saying it stopped getting better, though she was much improved and had returned to many of her prior activities. She remained at that level for three months, at which point I increased all of her dosages except Vitamin B12, which was kept at baseline because her fatigue was under control. Immediately, her condition began to improve again.

It took almost ten weeks before she could tolerate the recommended daily doses of Beta Carotene, complaining of nagging headaches that were relieved when she lowered her dosage; she had no problems with the other supplements.

After ten months on the daily supplements, Susan was ninety-five percent symptom free and had regained nearly all movement in previously effected joints. She was again running five miles a day along the ocean, and she took up roller blading with a vengeance. She had decreased her Tylenol intake to two tablets, once or twice a week. Though she was still taking the mild prescription anti-inflammatory, Susan had not taken any other arthritis drugs for a year when she visited her doctor for a complete work-up. He had not seen her for six months and was impressed with her recovery, writing in her medical chart, "However, it is good to see that she has gained marked symptomatic improvement during the interval months as she did not obtain relief with multiple other traditional medications used for rheumatoid arthritis. Perhaps the ... form of arthritis which she contracted after her illness in Mexico may prove responsive to the current vitamin and food supplement therapy which she is using."

EPILOGUE

Susan remained ninety-five percent symptom free from October 1995, until February 1997. For a six week period in 1996, she took no drugs whatsoever--not even Piroxicam or Tylenol--relying exclusively on supplements to control her disease. She decided to use Piroxicam again, because she could feel the difference without it. Then in 1997, her symptoms worsened, and she had to return to using gold injections. As of February 1999, she was still getting a weekly gold injection, though she has never had to return to the other array of drugs she used in the past.

Because her disease had not remained in remission, I did not think it fair to include the remedy in this text. Susan convinced me otherwise, pointing out that she has never been as sick as she was when she started the remedy--she still runs five miles a day when she has time away from her new job in sales. She knows the supplements are making a difference, because whenever she runs out and misses doses, her body's reaction is profoundly negative.

In her words, "Even if there is only one other person out there who will read this and be empowered to take their lives back the way I did, it will be worth it. I believe thousands will be helped by this remedy, but sometimes you can only help one person at a time. That doesn't make it any less important a thing to do."

CHAPTER 10

RUTIN

•Strengthen Blood Vessels And Prevent Their Rupture

Helping To Prevent Aneurism Stroke
Promoting Leg Vein Health And Preventing Varicose Veins
Avoiding Hemorrhoids
Stopping Bleeding Gums And Nosebleeds
Trading Bloodshot Eyes For Bright Eyes
Avoiding Ruptured Facial Capillaries
Preventing Leg Bruising If You Stand For Long Periods

Rutin is one of the nutrients found in Vitamin C Complex, which also contains Citrus Bioflavinoids, Hesperidin, and sometimes Acerola, in combination with Vitamin C. Taken in sufficient quantities, Rutin has an extraordinary ability to strengthen the walls of arteries, veins and capillaries, and can help prevent any disorder associated with weak blood vessels that rupture. Conditions responding to Rutin include brain ruptures leading to stroke, leg ruptures causing varicose veins, anal ruptures resulting in hemorrhoids, mouth and gum ruptures leading to bleeding gums, nasal cavity ruptures causing nosebleeds, whites-of-the-eye ruptures resulting in bloodshot eyes, facial ruptures that leave tiny spiderweb patterns across the nose, cheeks, and chin, and other ruptures that cause bruising.

All these conditions are due primarily to weak blood-vessel walls that rupture easily under the pressure within the arterial system, or from an exterior trauma such as a toothbrush injury or strong sneeze. Each can be a sign of a mild to serious Rutin deficiency and can become more pronounced when you drink, because alcohol destroys both Rutin and Vitamin C in your system.

Recommended Strength[24]

500 mg (You may use 1000 mg strength if you can find it. The author has been able to find high quality Rutin formulas only in the 500 mg size.)

Recommended Form

Tablets or capsules

Taken How

With eight ounces of juice or other liquids as directed.

Side Effects

None observed when taken as directed.

Notes√√

√ The elements of Vitamin C Complex, one of which is Rutin, work interactively. If you take Rutin on a long term basis, it is recommended that you also take **Vitamin C Complex**. Otherwise, you may deplete the other elements of the Complex and develop a different deficiency than the one you are treating. You do not have to take Vitamin C Complex and Rutin at the same time.

---

24 For Rutin the author has had the best results with Country Life®, Hauppauge, NY 11799, (800) 645-5768; Puritan's Pride®, Oakdale, NY 11769, (800) 645-1030; Solgar®, Leonia, NJ 07605, (800) 645-2246; and Twin Lab®, Ronkonkoma, NY 11779, (800) 645-5626. Puritan's Pride is available by mail order only. The other brands can be purchased at most health foods stores and sometimes in the health foods section of supermarkets.

Vitamin C Complex: Use in 1000 mg tablets or capsules. Take it with eight ounces of juice or other liquids as directed. The dosage strength is for Vitamin C only; the other trace components will be present in varying amounts depending upon the brand. You may use Vitamin C alone if you cannot find Vitamin C Complex.

1. Take 1000 mg twice daily, morning and evening, and continue as a maintenance dose as long as you take Rutin.

Remedy At A Glance (Vitamin C Complex)

Daily As A Maintenance Dose While Taking Rutin:	Morning	Evening
	1000 mg	1000 mg

See Chapter 3 for more on L-Cysteine and Vitamin C Complex and how to use the combination as a remedy for asthma and other respiratory disorders, to guard against cigarette smoker's damage, to prevent hangovers, to avoid liver/age spots, and to protect against environmental toxins.

See Chapter 7 for more on Bee Pollen and Vitamin C Complex and how to use the combination to heal colds, allergies, and sinus problems.

•Strengthen Blood Vessels And Prevent Their Rupture

Helping To Prevent Aneurism Stroke
Promoting Leg Vein Health And Preventing Varicose Veins
Avoiding Hemorrhoids

1. Take 2000 mg of Rutin four times daily, i.e., 8:00 a.m., noon, 4:00 p.m., and 8:00 p.m., and continue for four weeks.

2. Reduce to 2000 mg three times daily, morning, afternoon, and evening, and continue for four weeks.

3. Continue to take 1000 mg three times daily, morning, afternoon, and evening, as a maintenance dose to help prevent these conditions.

Remedy At A Glance (Rutin)

	8:00 am	Noon	4:00 pm	8:00 pm
Daily For Four Weeks To Relieve Symptoms:	2000 mg	2000 mg	2000 mg	2000 mg

	Morning	Afternoon	Evening
Daily For Four Weeks To Relieve Symptoms:	2000 mg	2000 mg	2000 mg
Daily As A Maintenance Dose:	1000 mg	1000 mg	1000 mg

Notes√√

√ This remedy can be very effective in helping prevent varicose veins in your legs, but it cannot remove them once they have ruptured and become visible. For that, cosmetic surgery is required. Ordinarily, this kind of ruptured blood vessel remains visible for the rest of your life--even more reason to try to prevent them.

√ This remedy can also be very effective in helping heal and prevent hemorrhoids. If your hemorrhoids are mild to moderate, the remedy can work in just days to bring complete relief. If you have a serious condition, one that is causing pain and substantial blood loss, you may need surgery to remove or seal the ruptured blood vessels. Be aware that blood in your stool can indicate a more serious condition, such as colon cancer, which may require medical attention. The Rutin remedy is designed for those who know they have hemorrhoids. It can bring strong relief, but *if your symptoms are severe you should consult a physician immediately.*

√ To help heal hemorrhoids, it is recommended that you also take **Beta Carotene**, because it accelerates healing anywhere in the body.

Beta Carotene: Use in 25,000 IU softgel form only. Take it once a day with your largest meal as directed, regardless of the amount you are taking.

1. Take 250,000 IU (10 softgels) daily, for the first two days of each week, i.e., Sunday and Monday.

2. Reduce to 200,000 IU (8 softgels) daily, for the next three days, i.e., Tuesday, Wednesday, and Thursday.

3. Reduce to 150,000 IU (6 softgels) daily, for the last two days, i.e., Friday and Saturday.

4. Follow this weekly schedule until your symptoms are gone, then reduce to 100,000 IU (4 softgels) daily, and continue for two weeks.

5. Continue to take 75,000 IU (3 softgels) daily, as a maintenance dose to help prevent hemorrhoids and promote health in soft tissue.

Remedy At A Glance (Beta Carotene)

	Once A Day With Largest Meal		
	Days 1-2	Days 3-5	Days 6-7
Daily To Relieve Symptoms:	250,000 IU	200,000 IU	150,000 IU
Daily For Two Weeks After You Are Better:	100,000 IU		
Daily As A Maintenance Dose:	75,000 IU		

See Chapter 5 for more on Beta Carotene and how to use it as a remedy to shorten healing time by more than half, and *drastically* reduce wound tenderness and scarring.

Stopping Bleeding Gums And Nosebleeds
Trading Bloodshot Eyes For Bright Eyes
Avoiding Ruptured Facial Capillaries
Preventing Leg Bruising If You Stand For
Long Periods

1. Take 2000 mg of Rutin four times daily, i.e., 8:00 a.m., noon, 4:00 p.m., and 8:00 p.m., and continue for three weeks.

2. Reduce to 2000 mg three times daily, morning, afternoon, and evening, and continue for three weeks.

3. Continue to take 1000 mg twice daily, morning and evening, as a maintenance dose to help prevent these conditions.

Remedy At A Glance (Rutin)

	8:00 am	Noon	4:00 pm	8:00 pm
Daily For Three Weeks To Relieve Symptoms:	2000 mg	2000 mg	2000 mg	2000 mg
	Morning	Afternoon	Evening	
Daily For Three Weeks To Relieve Symptoms:	2000 mg	2000 mg	2000 mg	
Daily As A Maintenance Dose:	1000 mg		1000 mg	.

Notes√√

√ This remedy can be very effective in helping prevent spider veins on your face, but it cannot remove them once they have ruptured and become visible. For that, cosmetic surgery is required. Facial spider ruptures can sometimes disappear when the remedy is begun *directly* after they appear. Ordinarily, this kind of ruptured blood vessel remains visible for the rest of your life--even more reason to try to prevent them.

√ Be aware that bleeding gums can also be a sign of other illness, such as gingivitis, which may require immediate dental attention. By preventing your gums from bleeding, Rutin could mask a more serious dental problem. In addition to taking Rutin, it is important to floss regularly and see your dentist twice a year for a check-up and cleaning. This routine will ensure that you catch any serious mouth and gum ailments early enough to treat them successfully.

*   *   *

The following is a case study written as a short story about one of the countless people who have been helped by this remedy: A Los Angeles "features model" having a really bad year uses Rutin to clear up at least one of his problems.

"Reality Check"

He parked the shiny-with-wax, black vintage 1964 Mustang, convertible top down, in Bally's Hollywood parking structure, grabbed his gym bag from the front seat as he was getting out, and activated the car alarm on his way into the club. Running his membership card through the scanner, he watched his name and particulars scroll across the computer screen: Jake N. O'Brien. Ht. 5' 8", Wt. 160 lbs. D.O.B. 4/8/62. N for Nicodemo. Giving a name to the Italian half would prevent it being lost inside the Irish, his mother said. Not a real possibility the way she'd raised Jake and his brother, Mitch. Surrounded by his father's large family--hers back in Palermo--she worried so about being absorbed into her husband's clan, losing her *Italianness*, that she overcompensated, making Macaulay O'Brien feel guilty if he so much as asked her to cook a pot of potato soup. The outcome being that even though Jake was encouraged in the O'Brien way, at his core he felt Italian. Mitch was the opposite, all about being Irish.

Jake headed for the lockers to deposit his gym bag and change clothes. Just outside the workout room he stepped on the scale. One seventy one. Jesus. Too much *Gnocchi Golosi* and *Vitello alla Valdostana* at Trattoria Cappolo with girlfriend, Diana. Before dinner scotches, two bottles of wine with the entrees, and dessert aperitifs upped the calorie count.

Both Jake and Diana were professional models in the unique position of not having to watch their weight. Not too much. Diana, a large-size model with a 5' 9" frame, nicely filled out size sixteen and ate whatever she wanted. Jake, homely with a high forehead, receding chin and Roman nose, made six-figures as a "features" model. Mostly hand and eye closeups. The back of his head was featured once in a popular men's hair coloring commercial still running in some TV markets, his black hair the after picture. You would have seen his green eyes in tight close-up, in magazine and TV ads, modeling eye glasses or trying to get the red out; watched them look tired in sleep remedy spots, and sick in cold and flu remedy ads. His manicured hands were on camera in one-in-five, hands-only print and TV ads produced in the last three years.

Hadn't been much work lately, but he knew down times were part of the business.

Jake ran fifteen minutes on the treadmill, keeping his heart rate around one hundred sixty beats per minute, for a good cardiac workout. Sweating hard, he followed it with fifteen minutes on the Stairmaster, making sure his heart rate now stayed between one twenty and one forty, the optimum rate for burning fat. He drank frequently from a liter bottle of Arrowhead spring water, glad he'd remembered to bring it. Stepping off the Stairmaster he entered an empty aerobics room and stretched for ten minutes. He lay on the floor, exhausted, thinking about blowing off the rest of the work out.

People began filtering in to the room for a body-sculpting class starting in ten minutes. They went directly to the storage wall to get their platforms, stretching rope, and hand weights, and then spread out to find a spot on the carpeted floor. Jake dragged himself up and out the door, wiping sweat that seemed to pour from his face and neck. On his way back to the machine room, he ran into his best friend and sometime workout partner, Rozzelle Brickman. Their fifteen-year friendship was back on after two years of not speaking, because Jake had caught Rosey in bed with his then girlfriend, Marla. But only after Rosey had caught Jake in bed with Corrine. Things were as even now as they would ever be.

Tall, black-skinned with a droopy Pancho Villa moustache and close-cropped hair, Rosey was a former Tuskegee running back headed for the first-round picks, until an injury in the last five minutes of the last game of the season tore apart his left knee. Looking closely, you could still detect a slight limp in his step, but he hung his shoulder into it, made it look on purpose. He taught Legal Research & The Computer, at Southwest Law School, six hours a week. Rest of the time he coached field sports at a private high school in Brentwood.

"Rosey, what up? Whatcha' doing man? Wanna' spot me?"

"Jake, my man. Sure thing, you'll return the favor." Rosey looking closely at Jake now, saying, "S--- man. You look terrible. What the hell happened to you? Haven't seen you here in a long-ass time neither."

Jake saying, "Nothin.' Nothing happened to me. What are you talking man? I don't know what the f--- you're talking about."

Rosey let it go.

For the next ninety minutes the men worked out individually on weight machines. Rosey, who alternated work out days, moved efficiently through exercises devoted to the upper body. Having no particular routine, Jake followed Rosey around the room, machine to machine. Jake knew Rosey concentrated hard when working out and didn't like to talk. But Rosey seemed more than a little preoccupied this morning, making Jake nervous, and he tried several times to start a conversation without success. First Rosey, then Jake, spent eight minutes each on five different machines to work forearms, biceps, pectorals, deltoids and triceps. Twenty minutes on a single machine designed to work the latissimus dorsi, lower back and obliques. Twenty-five minutes to keep the little boxes on the abs squared; Rosey's; Jake's were smooth as cheese. In the free weights room they spotted each other for another half hour. Jake pressing 90 pounds, Rosey 280. Jake spent another ten minutes back in an aerobics room stretching and warming down. Rosey went straight to the showers.

After showering, Jake found Rosey alone in the steam room, fourteen square feet of cedar. He was stretched out naked on the wooden slats, white towel under his head as a pillow, arms resting at his side, looking like he was asleep. Jake, wearing a navy towel wrapped around his waist, kept himself covered as he sat down against the near wall. Trying to forget what he'd just heard in the showers. Jesus. Deal with it later.

Three Asian men, tanned, white haired and bony, entered the hot moist room wrapped in white towels that covered them from shoulder to mid calf. They sat down against the far wall, speaking

187

rapidly in their own language, sounding just short of an argument, and paying no attention to Jake or Rosey.

After a few minutes, Rosey opened his eyes and moved his right arm behind his head. He liked the steam room, felt good on his bum knee. Pausing to get it right, he said to Jake, "Word going around is you're into Johnny Maple for over 15K." He said, "Now everybody knows Maple is no wise guy. But he don't like you stiffing him. Looking to sell your markers to somebody won't be so patient, understanding. Thought you gave up gambling anyway, Jake. You ain't no good at it."

Thinking Rosey was asleep, and lulled by the heat and the incomprehensible singsong voices of the men at the other end of the room, Jake had dozed off. When Rosey started talking he had to go back to grab the beginning, see what it was he said.

"The f--- you telling me? How in hell would you know?" Jake sounding surprised and a little scared.

Rosey waited. Giving it time to sink in. S---. Couldn't be *that* big a surprise. Think the man was going to wait forever for his money?

"Had dinner with Michelle, works for Maple. Remember her? Smart sister, short blonde afro, big ones? Yeah. Said Maple's thinking of retiring. Anyway, wants to tie up loose ends. You a major loose end, man."

Calmer now, Jake said, "You did more'n have dinner, she told you that."

Rosey ignored the remark. Draping the white towel around his neck and shoulders, hanging on to each end with a closed fist, he stood and walked to the door, saying, "Maybe you'll get lucky, they'll only kick your ass. Won't break your fingers, put out an eye, keep you from making a living."

The glass door closed silently in the face of the escaping steam. Jake leaned back against the wood and thought about Rosey's words. Christ! He was getting screwed all over the place, first the showers now the steam room.

*   *   *

In a Santa Monica restaurant a waiter led Jake to a table on the terrace overlooking the Pacific Ocean, where Diana was enjoying a glass of Chablis and a charbroiled Ichiban appetizer. The incoming tide had saturated the air with brine scent. After pecking her full lips, he accepted a mouthful of the delicate fish she offered on a fork tip. A soft breeze stirred the thick, black hair spilling over her brown shoulders. She wore a sleeveless aqua jumpsuit with white belt; white jacket hanging over the back of the chair; white sandals showing pampered feet and manicured toenails, painted navy to match her fingernails. Jake thinking she looked good enough to be on the menu.

Diana wiped her mouth on a napkin and flashed her "beautiful model" smile. Telling Jake she was still in character and had something unpleasant to say. Jesus, what else? Her Mexican sensibilities would keep it until after they'd eaten, would give him the solace of a full stomach. Jake signaled the waiter and ordered a double scotch, prime rib, garlic mashed potatoes, and tossed salad with blue cheese dressing. Reaching for the still warm sourdough bread, he tore off and buttered a fist-sized chunk, only half listening to Diana telling him about her catalogue shoot that afternoon. Rosey's words still in his ears, distracting him. Fifteen thousand! More even. Jesus.

Interrupting her, Jake asked, "Were you able to get any blow?"

Chewing with her mouth full, Diana only nodded. She swallowed, placed a napkin to her mouth, and sipped wine before saying, "Don't know why you going there again, Jake." Voice soft, without accusation. "You were clean how long? Two years? You start up with this crap again six months ago. You don't need this. I'm telling you, you don't."

They didn't talk much after that. Dinner conversation was mostly about the food, which was good. Diana ordering more wine. Jake drinking double scotches. When the dishes were cleared and the credit voucher signed, Diana reached across the table. "Maybe you *should* get a buzz on before we go to the movie. I have bad news," she said, sounding apologetic.

Jake accepted the tiny glass vial in his palm without responding, told Diana he would meet her outside at valet parking, and headed for the men's room.

Standing outside waiting for Jake, mentally kicking herself, Diana swore it was the last time she would let him talk her into this s---. She didn't use drugs, so why should she be scoring for someone else? Just because she could? She knew there was a nasty name for people like her. Enabler.

189

*   *   *

Jake drove south on Lincoln Boulevard, then east on Venice, looking for the Beaux Arts, a frumpy little movie theatre that just opened last month and would be closed within the year. Offered second runs of popular movies for three bucks a person. Currently showing *Thelma & Louise*, Diana's favorite. She owned two copies of the video, watched it once a week, but still wanted to see it again on the big screen.

"You want to tell me about losing the Monet account you're too late," Jake said. "Heard it from Spears this morning at the club. In the f---ing shower no less."

He kept quiet about what Rosey told him in the steam room.

Diana sucked in her breath and said, "You lost Olgivy?"

"Just the Monet eye glass account ...." If she didn't want to tell him about Monet what the hell did she have to say? Christ! he'd be glad when this day was over.

Diana turned on the radio, scanning the buttons for a light jazz station.

Here it comes he thought.

The silence lasted two more traffic lights before she said at the end of a deep sigh, "Coca Cola isn't going to use you on this summer's shoot. Jim Mercury's casting. He was at my shoot this afternoon. So was your agent. I overheard them talking." Diana reached out to take Jake's right hand, resting lightly on the gearshift. He moved it to grip the steering wheel, knuckles white.

"Spears *told* you that? The f--- is happening? My own agent?

Diana interrupted him, "I told you I overheard it."

"Why didn't he just say something this morning when he told me Monet dumped me. In the f---ing shower."

"Probably didn't know it then," Diana said. "The shoot ran until after six. Spears and Mercury left together around five."

"I've had Coca-Cola for six years. Why would they suddenly dump me?"

"Are you kidding?" she asked. When Jake only stared ahead, eyes blank, she said, "Could it be that last year production ran over two days because you kept arguing with the director? Wouldn't do what you was told. All she ask you for is do the close-up facing the fountain ...."

190

Jake interrupted her, "My hands look chubby from that angle. We always do it stage right. Why suddenly change? Ask me, the chick wanted to try something new just to be different."

"She's not allowed to try something new she wants to? *Coca Cola* for God's sake. Either way, wasn't your business. You weren't directing, she was."

The silence lasted five traffic lights until Jake said, "I'm in no mood to see a movie. Sure as hell don't want to see f---ing *Thelma and Louise* again."

"What'sa matter, Jake? Can't stand a movie where women doing what they want, not what they told?"

*   *   *

At his front door Jake thought about Diana, about driving back down to her place. Show up with flowers, sweep her off her feet--maybe take her to the marina and spend the night on the boat. He shelved the idea because there was no place close to buy flowers. Couldn't risk the chance Irma might show up at the boat looking for him, either. And he needed gas. He unlocked the door and picked up the mail sprawled on the floor just inside. One envelope with Spears' logo caught his eye. He tore it open as he headed for the kitchen to get a drink. He didn't read past the first sentence--*We regret to inform you that CTC will not be exercising their two-year option*--before crumpling the letter and tossing it across the room.

What was happening? Just a year ago, seemed like he turned down two, maybe three, jobs a month.

Jake went into the bathroom, washed his hands and splashed cold water on his face. After drying himself on a towel he studied his reflection in the mirror, holding his face close to the glass. Right eye had a big 'ol red smudge right next to the iris, which looked dull and washed-out; whites shot through with tiny red lines, Jesus! making him look ten years older. He turned away from the mirror to find the phone and call Spears again, then changed his mind and dialed Chicago. "Hi Mom, it's me," he said into the receiver.

*   *   *

Going south on the San Diego Freeway out of Los Angeles, Jake followed Interstate 5 into Mission Viejo, where he stopped for breakfast: two Egg McMuffins and an apple turnover. He sat at a table sipping black coffee on an outdoor patio facing the mall parking lot, only half full this early. Thinking, as he wiped his mouth on a paper napkin, that like most agents Spears was full of s---. Didn't know what he was doing half the time. Like Jake was some amateur who would get a hard on because Spears had bad news for him. What? Because he lost his temper that one time last year and broke a few things? One time was enough to change a person's whole attitude about you? Spears was the amateur, not Jake. But that's what Spears called Jake right before telling him that he screwed up the job in San Diego, he was finished with the agency. Hey, no problem. It was only catalogue work--jewelry, a piece of cake--but good money, free hotel room and expenses. A free watch in it too, maybe score gold cufflinks and a chain. Jake didn't want to push Spears too far, still needed the a--hole, for now. He got hot again he'd sign with another agency fast. Anyway, be nice to get the hell out of L.A. for two weeks.

An hour later Jake checked into The Town and Country in Mission Valley's Hotel Circle, fifteen minutes northeast of downtown San Diego. It had a large pool, a coffee shop where the smell of frying bacon made Jake think he was hungry when he walked by, and a large convention center where the catalogue would be shot. Bally's Fitness was on the other side of the highway, and it was a short drive to Ocean Beach and the mighty Pacific. Not too shabby.

*　　　*　　　*

Hard as I've tried, I have never been able to find a substitute for exercise and its benefits of low weight and good health. I cross train: walk/run along San Diego's Mission Bay two or three times a week, racking up about ten miles, visit Bally's Mission Valley once or twice a week, and work out at home to the first *Buns Of Steel* tape with Greg Smithey--a real butt toner and hip tamer. I usually start each session at Bally's with the intention of doing a half-hour on the Stairmaster in the large downstairs room, but often, after only fifteen minutes I'm upstairs in the smaller women-preferred workout room, hefting machine weights, telling myself I get good cardiac workouts on my runs along the bay. This particular morning I made it through the half hour and decided to stay downstairs to try a new machine not available upstairs, one that simulated chin-ups. I wanted to gain more upper body strength, though my shoulders and arms had already forced me from a size small to a medium.

Not wearing my contacts or glasses I had to stand close to the machine to read the instructions. I could hear metal weights clanging to a rest, the whir of Stairmasters and treadmills, and the swoosh of hydraulic equipment, all overlaid by music from a local radio station playing hits from the eighties and nineties. Earth, Wind, & Fire were doing "Hearts of Fire." Before I could finish reading and digest the information, a voice said over my shoulder, "I can show you how you need some help."

Turning around slightly, not all the way, I said, "Thanks, I can read."

I finished on that machine and headed for the juice bar before going upstairs for the rest of my workout. Downstairs is four times larger, noisy, and stocked with mostly newer, hydraulic equipment. I liked the relative quiet upstairs and preferred the clean, fluid feel of moving steel against gravity. The juice was freshly squeezed from oranges stacked in a shallow bin along the back wall. It tasted wonderful, deep orange in color and sugar sweet. I listened to the music overhead: Maxi Priest, the seducer, singing,"I Just Wanna Be Close To You." *To do all the things you want me to.* To my left I watched a row of glass-enclosures, where several men--two to a room--played racquet ball, really going at it. They looked good with muscles pumped and sweaty t-shirts sticking to their chests and backs.

I sipped my juice, and heard the same voice from behind again, saying, "I didn't mean anything in there. Just wanted to help out."

I turned around smiling, saying it was ok.

*   *   *

Jake noticed her while she was on the Stairmaster, exaggerating each step, like she was lazy and didn't really want to do it. Moving her hips side to side in time to the music, James Brown's, "Hot Pants." About his height and age, he thought. Thinner than he liked--maybe size eight or ten, but nice anyway. Real nice. Brown skin that looked soft to touch. He watched her leave the workout room and followed. Hell the ice was broken now. They'd already had a conversation of sorts. Owed her an apology at least. He'd be cool about it. Wouldn't push it. Was going to be in San Diego another ten days. Diana couldn't leave L.A. Be nice to have some company.

When she turned around he started to say something about her smile, but something familiar stopped him. Then he knew and said her name, "Lynn," his voice flat but with a trace of wonder.

*   *   *

Walking across the parking lot on our way to TGI Friday's for lunch at Jake's invitation, he said for the fourth time, "Jesus, you look great. Haven't changed at all. What's it been, ten years? No eleven. Summer of 1985 right? You were still in law school, clerking at some New York firm."

"Thanks, you haven't changed either," I lied.

"Sure, that's why you had so much trouble recognizing me." Smiling easy when he said it, not taking offense. Still teasing he asked, "When's the last time you spoke to my big brother? You know, no one's allowed to say your name around Mitch he don't give 'em s--- about it. After all this time."

"The feeling's mutual so maybe we should talk about something else."

"I told you back then you were with the wrong O'Brien."

I smiled and let it go as we entered Friday's foyer, where benches stood against two walls and a four-foot gum machine occupied the center.

"I heard you got a divorce," he said. "I'm in a serious two year relationship myself, with a beautiful woman. Diana Morales. We're thinking about getting married."

"That why you were hitting on me?"

"I wasn't hitting on you. Just trying to help is all."

"Are you faithful to Diana?"

Jake shrugged, saying, "Mostly," as he sat down across from me at a table next to a large window. Full sun warmed the red-and-white checkered tablecloth and felt nice in the air-cooled atmosphere. Fresh cooked--still warm--corn chips and salsa were placed on the table shortly after we sat down. We shared a spinach salad for two with hot

194

dressing and huge tender prawns. Jake selected an oak flavored Chardonnay and encouraged me to tell him about my marriage, divorce, and new book, while we ate.

He said, "I'm trying to understand why you went to law school so you could come out and write medical books."

"It's not exactly a medical book."

"It's not a *law* book."

"It's a long story." I dropped my napkin on the tablecloth, saying, "Your turn, Jake. Tell me about yourself. Heard you were a big-time model on television, doing commercials." I was looking at his face, wondering how he'd managed that.

As if reading my mind, he said, "I know I look like hell now." Then after a pause, "I let myself go on purpose. I wanted some time off and the phone kept ringing."

I just looked at him.

"That's a joke," he said, before telling me about the past couple of months, ending with the day he lost three accounts and was threatened by a bookie. I think it was easy for him to talk to me. We shared common history, but he knew I wouldn't be around in the future.

He drained his wine glass, saying, "Got anything in that book'll fix my bloodshot eyes?"

"Sure thing. Chapter ten, Rutin."

"Never heard of it," he said, signaling the waiter for a scotch and soda. "How long will it take to work? Do I need a prescription?"

"These are *food* supplements, Jake. No prescriptions needed. Takes just a few days, maybe a week. Help if you stopped drinking so much."

"What makes you think I drink too much? Shared one bottle of white wine with you. Ordered my first scotch just a minute ago."

"Besides your bloodshot eyes? You're getting a nose like W.C. Fields, tiny broken blood vessels. That's often a sign you're tossing 'em back plenty." I pantomimed taking a drink.

Jake looked hurt but shrugged it off, being cool. "I don't drink that much. No way," he said, and remembered the face he'd examined in the mirror recently. "Maybe wouldn't hurt to try your remedy, I guess. What have I got to lose?"

He wrote the instructions for the six-week regimen on a paper napkin, while we shared a huge slice of mud pie covered with melted chocolate.

*   *   *

Jake called me a few days before leaving town to tell me how well the remedy worked. "It's real nice. Been taking extra when I drink, like you told me. Pretty impressive, way it works. Going to take it all the time."

"Good. I'm really happy. Don't forget the Vitamin C."

"I remember, Vitamin C *Complex*, I wrote it down. Bought 'em both."

"Maybe I'll use you in my book."

"Only if I can share the royalties," he said, and laughed. "There was one other thing. I'm gonna be here for another couple of days ... ahh."

"Jake, I'm sorry. I'm not interested."

"Let me finish, you don't understand. I wondered if you could tell me where ... you know, an AA meeting in the area? You said your ex-husband .... Thought I'd stop by, give the program another chance. Haven't been in a couple of months."

"Does this mean you're going to stop drinking?" I asked.

"Probably. I don't know. Maybe. Yeah."

CHAPTER 11

VITAMIN B12

•Combat Short-Term Fatigue And Low Energy
Gaining More Energy Within Hours

•Stop Tingling Extremities
Improving Overall Circulation

Vitamin B12, also known as cobalamin concentrate, is one of the components of Vitamin B Complex, which also includes B1 (Thiamin), B2 (Riboflavin), B3 (Niacin), B5 (Pantothenic Acid), B6 (Pyridoxine), PABA (Para-Aminobenzoic Acid), Folic Acid, and Biotin. B12 is the only one of these elements that cannot be synthesized in a laboratory or extracted from plants like other supplements, but must be grown in bacteria or molds like penicillin. It is also the only one that cannot be obtained from a variety of food sources. It is found only in red meat, dairy products, or by taking it in supplement form--so vegetarian diets provide little or no B12. Since most people are eating less red meat and dairy products, in an attempt to lower cholesterol, a B12 deficiency is more likely to occur today.

A primary role of Vitamin B12, essential for the formation of red blood cells, is the efficient transport of oxygen to all parts of the body. Fatigue is an immediate result of insufficient quantities of B12. Taken in supplement form, it can work fast--within hours of the first dose--to relieve fatigue and provide a sustained energy level throughout the day.

Another sign that can indicate a deficiency is tingling extremities--legs, feet, arms, and fingers, that "go to sleep" when you are still for a period of time. Vitamin B12 can help ensure that more oxygen-rich blood is available when you need it anywhere in you body.

Recommended Strength[25]

1000 mcg

Recommended Form

Tablets, capsules, or sublingual

Taken How

With eight ounces of juice or other liquids as directed. (Sublingual is dissolved under the tongue and requires no liquid.)

Side Effects

None observed when taken as directed.

Notes√√

√ If you take Vitamin B12 for more than a few days at a time, it is recommended that you also take **Vitamin B Complex**, to avoid depleting other elements of the B Complex and causing a different deficiency than the one you are treating. You do not have to take B Complex and B12 together--at the same time. Be aware that B Complex can turn urine a darker yellow due to the concentration of nutrients present in B vitamins, and this is not cause for alarm.

---

25 Since Vitamin B12 can be synthesized only one way, most brands are comparable. Try to avoid brands that use a large number of fillers and "other ingredients." Time-released or sustained-release products are *not* recommended.

Vitamin B Complex: Use B Complex 100, tablets or capsules.[26] (Some B vitamins included in the 100 complex are measured in milligrams, others in micrograms, but all will be contained in one tablet or capsule.) Vitamin B Complex is available in higher strength formulas, up to B Complex 150, and you may use a higher strength formula if you wish. Take it with food, because it can be hard to digest.

1. Take one tablet or capsule once a day, and continue as a maintenance dose as long as you take Vitamin B12.

Remedy At A Glance (Vitamin B Complex)

Daily As A Maintenance Dose While Taking B12:	Once A Day With Food
	B Complex 100 or higher

See Volume II of this series for more on Vitamin B Complex and how to use it as a remedy for certain kinds of nervousness, including muscle tics and trembling in your extremities.

•Combat Short-Term Fatigue And Low Energy

Gaining More Energy Within Hours

1. Take 2000 mcg of Vitamin B12 twice daily, morning and early afternoon, and continue for two weeks.

2. Reduce to 2000 mcg in the morning, 1000 mcg in the early afternoon, and continue as a maintenance dose to help maintain your

---

26 For Vitamin B Complex, the author has had the best results with Country Life®, Hauppauge, NY 11788, (800) 645-5768; Puritan's Pride®, Oakdale, NY 11769, (800) 645-1030; and Solgar®, Leonia, NJ 07605, (800) 645-2246. Puritan's Pride is available by mail order only. The other brands can be purchased at most health foods stores and sometimes in the health foods section of supermarkets.

increased energy levels.

Remedy At A Glance (Vitamin B12)

	Morning	Early Afternoon
Daily For Two Weeks To Relieve Symptoms:	2000 mcg	2000 mcg
Daily As A Maintenance Dose:	2000 mcg	1000 mcg

See Chapter 6 for Coenzyme Q10 and how to use it as a remedy to help alleviate long-term fatigue and increase endurance.

Notes√√

√ If Vitamin B12 does not work for you, it may indicate that your digestive system does not produce one of the gastric secretions necessary to absorb it when taken orally. If so, you can use the sublingual form, which is dissolved under your tongue and absorbed directly into your bloodstream, bypassing the intestinal tract. You can also obtain B12 shots from your physician.

√ Your fatigue may stem from an Iron deficiency anemia, and you will need a blood test to find this out. If you are anemic, it is recommended that you add **Iron** to Vitamin B12.

Iron: Use 15 mg tablets from ferrous gluconate, which is generally easier to digest than ferrous sulfate.[27] Take it once a day with food. It can take approximately four weeks for your body to synthesize the supplements and make enough new blood cells to raise your red blood cell count.

1. Take 15 mg daily, and continue as long as your red blood cell count is below normal: 12 to 14 for women, and 14 to 16 for men.

---

[27] There are too many quality brands available to mention here. Try to buy one that does not use fillers and a lot of "other ingredients."

2. When your red blood cell count has returned to normal, reduce to 15 mg every other day, and continue as a maintenance dose to avoid anemia.

3. Before you take Iron supplements, be sure you do not have a genetic condition called hemochromatosis, which causes you to absorb too much Iron from food (seventy-five percent instead of the average ten to fifteen percent). The excess Iron can actually start to rust inside your body and can be very toxic.

Remedy At A Glance (Iron)

	Once A Day With Food
Daily To Raise Red Blood Cell Count:	15 mg
Every Other Day As A Maintenance Dose:	15 mg

See Volume II of this series for more on Iron and how to use it to treat anemia and fatigue.

If you experience constipation while taking Iron, see Chapter 12 for information on how to use Magnesium Oxide to help prevent it.

√ The B12 remedy is a baseline treatment for fatigue and low energy and is meant to be taken on a regular basis. If you experience fatigue only occasionally--under specific conditions, or at certain times --you may wish to use B12 only then. Here are a few tips:

To Relieve Morning Fatigue: If you go to bed tired, facing an early morning wake up, and knowing you will not get enough sleep--or if you usually have trouble getting up in the morning--this method can make it easier to wake up, feel good, and be alert from the start of the day. This procedure can also be effective during school exams, caring for a newborn, law enforcement stakeouts, and other times when you get little or no sleep for an extended period.

1. Take 2000 mcg sixty seconds before bed. If too much time elapses between taking B12 and going to bed, sleep may be disturbed.

2. Take 2000 mcg as soon as you wake up.

Remedy At A Glance (Vitamin B12)

	Directly Before Bed	As Soon As You Wake Up
To Relieve Morning Fatigue:	2000 mcg	2000 mcg

To Relieve Afternoon Fatigue: If you experience a midday energy slump--usually occurring an hour after eating lunch--when you have an almost irresistible desire to nap, B12 can eliminate drowsiness and help you maintain high levels of energy to stay alert through the rest of the day.

1. Take 2000 mcg two hours before lunch.

2. Take 2000 mcg directly after you eat.

Remedy At A Glance (Vitamin B12)

	Two Hours Before Lunch	Directly After You Eat
To Relieve Afternoon Fatigue:	2000 mcg	2000 mcg

To Relieve Evening Fatigue: If you find yourself nodding off in the early evening and missing precious time with your family or work on a favorite project, B12 can prevent evening drowsiness and add extra hours to your day, permitting you to accomplish more.

1. Take 2000 mcg at noon, and 2000 mcg an hour before dinner. If you do not eat dinner, take it no later than 5:00 p.m.

2. Be aware that taking B12 in the latter part of the day can disturb your sleep that night. If this happens, take the second dose

earlier in the day.

Remedy At A Glance (Vitamin B12)

	Noon	One Hour Before Dinner
To Relieve Evening Fatigue:	2000 mcg	2000 mcg

•Stop Tingling Extremities

Improving Overall Circulation

1. Take 2000 mcg of Vitamin B12 in the morning, and 2000 mcg in the afternoon.

2. Take 1000 mcg before dinner. If you do not eat dinner, take it no later than 5:00 p.m.

3. Continue at this level until your symptoms are gone.

4. Reduce to 2000 mcg twice daily, morning and afternoon, and continue as a maintenance dose to help prevent tingling extremities.

Remedy At A Glance (Vitamin B12)

	Morning	Afternoon	Evening
Daily To Relieve Symptoms:	2000 mcg	2000 mcg	1000 mcg
Daily As A Maintenance Dose:	2000 mcg	2000 mcg	

Notes√√

√ Be aware that tingling extremities can also be an indication of other serious illnesses that may require immediate medical attention. *If your symptoms are severe you should consult a physician immediately.*

*   *   *

The following is a case study written as a short study about one of the countless people who have been helped by this remedy. A ninety-two year old granddaughter of a slave gets an energy boost from B12 to outpace her forty-something nephew at San Diego's Sea World.

"Sisters"

1924
Carlisle, Pennsylvania

Truth be known, Betsy never cared a whit for all the attention men paid her. Surrounded now by a group of bachelors on the porch steps of her father's drug store, she felt Nan watching her from the swing in the front yard. Nan was always watching, like an understudy who hoped to take over her sister's role some day. Watching the way Betsy tilted her head back when she laughed, noting the sound of it, high and carefree. Watching how she swung her crossed leg back and forth, sometimes touching the leg of the man seated closest to her, letting it linger there before swinging back. How she slouched thin shoulders to lean close and whisper something intimate in another's ear.

From the house next door, the jazz strains of "King Porter Stomp," by Jelly Roll Morton, were coming from a radio console occupying the front corner of the living room. Betsy looked casually toward her baby sister and motioned with one hand for her to join them. Nan pretended not to notice, turning her head to watch after-dinner strollers and the occasional Model T chugging down Main Street. Fireflies glittered yellow-orange in the deepening blue-violet twilight, and a warm wind sailed through the tops of chestnut trees, carrying the calls of the night.

Born three years apart, the sisters--Betsy and Nan--looked like they came from different families: Betsy was five feet two inches, lean and strong bodied, with a hardy constitution and skin the color of a sun-dried raisin. Dark velvety hair had been cut into a short bob in time for her twenty-second birthday. Her eyes were shiny black coals, and her broad features a fusion of the African and Indian blood lines from their

204

mother's side of the family.

At five feet seven inches, Nan was big boned, but frail and sickly, with skin the color of french vanilla ice cream and green eyes that sometimes looked blue. Auburn hair was braided in two plaits pinned together across the top of her head, and her features told of the African and Irish mixture acquired from their father's side. Childhood diseases had regularly confined Nan to her bed. When they ran their course, she was taken down with colds or flu, and twice with pneumonia. Sometimes her parents knew what was wrong, sometimes they didn't. She missed a lot of school and graduated thanks to Betsy's home lessons.

At the birthday party earlier that day, Betsy's parents gave her a 1921 Pierce-Arrow two passenger runabout, her first car and a real treasure since half the cars on the road were Ford's Model T. It would take her to Virginia in September where she would study business administration and accounting at Hampton Institute. The runabout was sleek and luxurious, egg-yolk yellow, with low-slung styling that added to its roadability. The seats were thickly cushioned tan leather. Betsy had been driving since she was fifteen; Nan didn't want to learn.

World War I had ended six years earlier. Calvin Coolidge, the thirtieth president, was in office. Susan B. Anthony had spearheaded the women's suffrage movement helping American women win the right to vote in 1920, with the passage of the Nineteenth Amendment, the same year the League of Nations was formed; the 1922 elections were the first time women voted. African-Americans were still referred to as Negroes, colored, and worse, and in the southeast, lynchings and burnings of black men were common. Still, many blacks prospered thanks to their own initiative--and that of their forbears--along with government post civil war reconstruction efforts.

Betsy and Nan were sheltered from the worst pains of segregation because of the family's money and position in the community. Their mother's father, Abelman Hadley, had won his freedom well before other slaves in 1863, and fought for the Union. His leg was shot off in '66 in the Memphis Massacre, when a mob attacked fifty black soldiers, killing most of them. He had trouble getting around after that and built the drugstore up from a small roadside stand where he sold hard candy, fruits, and homemade elixirs. Betsy and Nan's parents met and married shortly after their father was hired to set up the store's first pharmacy in 1900.

Betsy headed down the sloping lawn toward her sister, trailed by her five-man entourage. The wind pushed against her lavender dress, cut in the straight line drop-waist style of the flappers, camouflaging the body and emphasizing comfort.

Betsy said, "Hey Poodle, we're taking a ride in the new car. Going over to Harrisburg for ice cream. Come on along why don't you?"

"It's getting dark. Papa says it's not safe to drive at night. Does he know what you're planning?" Nan wore a pained expression and one of their mother's square-shoulder dresses passed down to her.

"That's why we have lanterns on the front. One for each side of the road," Betsy said, and her gentlemen callers laughed together as if cued by a conductor.

Betsy reached for Nan's hand, but she resisted. "Why do you want to drive all the way to Harrisburg when Papa has ice cream just inside?"

"All the way, kiddo? Only eighteen miles. We're doing it for the thrill, the excitement of the open road. The runabout can go *seventy* miles an hour. Why, it's practically like flying! Besides, Papa only carries vanilla, chocolate, and strawberry. Harrisburg has a place that scoops up exotic flavors like blueberry, bing cherry, raspberry, coffee, and orange sherbet."

"I don't think I want to go."

"Come on, live a little," Betsy said, taking Nan's hand and pulling her out of the swing.

Nan got in the passenger side, Betsy took the wheel. Two of the men declined the trip and said good night. The others followed in a Model T. Betsy pulled away from the curb and straightened the wheel before opening a leather flask to take a swig. Prohibition was in its fifth year, but hadn't stopped anyone from drinking. Millions of gallons of alcohol were sold legally each year under the Volsted Act, which permitted a druggist to sell it for medicinal purposes if prescribed by a doctor. Their father didn't notice Betsy's pilfering; if he did he kept it to himself.

"Aww, you oughtn't to do that Bet," Nan warned.

"Improves my driving. Here, try some."

Nan took the flask, the leather feeling warm in her hand, tilted it to her mouth and choked down a small gulp, which sent shivers up her back and through her stomach, raising bumps along her arms. The warmth spreading in her chest felt good.

She turned to smile at Betsy who was staring at the road ahead with a look of sheer pleasure on her face. "You always take care of me don't you, Bet?"

"Sure thing, Poodle. And I always will."

1960
Harlem, New York

"Beautiful service, Poodle, Harold would've been proud. Laid him out real nice," Betsy said. The sisters were riding in a black limousine on their way back to St. Helena Funeral Home, after a graveside service for Nan's husband. Betsy wore a black knit tube dress with a hood that covered her head, and a three-strand pearl necklace. Nan wore a black shirtwaist, no jewelry. Her black wide-brimmed hat had a veil that was pinned away from her face. On the seat between them was James Baldwin's, *Notes Of A Native Son*; Betsy intended to read it on the plane.

"He was a good man. Gave me two lovely children. A good man. Took care of me for thirty years. Took care of us all. Yes, Lord. We had *so* many plans .... " Nan's voice broke. "He was retiring next year, did I tell you? Thirty years with the railroad. Was going to take me to Europe." She started to cry.

Betsy moved closer and rubbed Nan's back. She sighed and said, "Come on, Poodle. Harold was a bastard. You and I both know that. And Europe isn't what it's cracked up to be. Too damp."

Nan sat up and pulled away from Betsy's embrace. "What are you saying?"

"About Europe?"

"About my dead husband."

"You heard me. He beat you senseless on more occasions than I care to remember. He was a lush. He was unfaithful. Has two illegitimate children I know about, probably more I don't. You're better off without him."

"He was a good businessman and provider," Nan protested. "Left six rentals to support me in my old age." Talking louder now.

207

"Worked almost every day of his life from the time he was six. How you can talk about him like that, I don't know."

"I say anything *wasn't* true?" Betsy insisted.

"You've never been married, Bet. You don't know the bond that forms and grows between a husband and wife. You've had financial success, a career, yes, but you've never had the tie that binds. Praise the Lord."

Betsy shrugged as if it didn't matter, as if the remark hadn't hit home, when it was a sore point on which she still second guessed herself. Eddie's face popped into her mind and she desperately wanted to change the subject. "One thing I do know is you can't run those six rentals."

"What's your point?"

"Either get one of those worthless sons of yours to take on the responsibility, or sell them and move out to San Diego with me. Weather on the East Coast stinks," Betsy said, sounding harsher than she meant to, still stinging from Nan's words.

Nan stared at Betsy while she wiped her eyes with a pink handkerchief. She emptied her nose and said, "You haven't changed a bit, not in all these years. You say and do whatever you want without any regard to another person's feelings. Well, if you say one more word about my children I will slap you silly. I swear I will."

"Calm down," Betsy said, and lighted a Benson & Hedges cigarette.

They were going south on St. Nicholas Avenue in Morningside Heights, rolling to a stop at a traffic light at 145th Street. The sky was overcast and hanging close; a light drizzle pattered the windows. Muffled music from another car stopped at the light came into the limo despite its closed windows; it was a Chuck Berry cut, though Betsy couldn't name the song. A small newspaper stand painted dark green sat on the corner. Betsy blew out cigarette smoke and studied the headlines on the displayed newspapers until the light changed:

DEMOCRATS PICK KENNEDY & JOHNSON

NEHRU SPEAKS AT UNITED NATIONS

COLD WAR OF WORDS: THREATS FLY BETWEEN VP

Betsy finished the cigarette and stubbed it in the ashtray on the door, saying, "I'm sorry Nan. You're right. I've lived for myself and my career all these years. Don't know what it means to have a family to worry about and take care of. Will you accept my apology?"

Nan took her hand. "Of course I will, Bet." They shifted slightly as the limo turned left on 135th Street heading for the east side.

"I still want you to think seriously about coming out to San Diego. There's plenty of land, it's still cheap. Build you a nice house overlooking the ocean, orange grove in the back yard. How about it, Poodle? The men are hotter in southern California."

"You're wicked," Nan said, and let go of Betsy's hand. "We aren't school girls anymore, you know. I'm fifty-four. You can't control me and tell me what to do."

"I know that. But I've been looking out for you too long to stop now. You can't teach an old dog new tricks."

The limousine stopped in front of St. Helena. Nan gathered herself to leave, body language showing her discomfort, saying she was already some place else.

"Will you at least think about it? About moving to the West Coast? Be easier to pull off than you think."

The driver got out and walked around to open the back door on the curbside. The sisters hugged, then Nan accepted the driver's hand in getting out.

She turned back and said through the open door, "The brownstone'll be lonely without Harold. All the children gone. I'll think about it. That's all I'll promise."

"Good enough, Poodle, take care."

The driver shut the door and returned to the front seat. He continued south to 125th Street, then east to the Triboro Bridge and Queens, to drop Betsy at La Guardia for her four o'clock flight on Pan American.

1994
San Diego, California

Betsy waited for the wheelchair van at the entrance ramp to Cedar Hills Convalescent Home, near the Sharp Memorial Hospital

209

Complex. She leaned lightly on the carved ebony cane she carried to steady herself when her knees gave. Her back was straight though her shoulders hunched a bit. She was wearing grey cotton slacks and a white blouse with a white cardigan over her shoulders, that stood out next to her dark skin. Her blue-and-white Nikes made her feet look too large for her small, lean frame. Her hair had greyed but was still bobbed short, hugging her face. She had most of her teeth and didn't wear glasses except to read. More importantly, the eyes that were black coals still shone with vitality and clarity.

With her free hand Betsy held Muffin's leash, the six-year-old long-coat Chihuahua waiting patiently at her feet. A baby-blue ribbon tied between her ears bobbed as the dog darted her head, tracking a large fly. Without notice Betsy studied the solemn little group standing with her: Nan's only grandson Chase, and his second wife Vashti, wearing matching Banana Republic safari suits that stopped at the knee. And her dear friend and neighbor Harvey, dressed like, well, like Harvey. At forty-five Chase was the same little whiner he'd been as a child. Always a tattler, he could be counted on to sell out to grown-ups for a promise of immunity. He was a lawyer in Oakland. Vashti was fifteen years his junior and ran her own accounting firm. She almost never talked as far as Betsy could tell. They were both about as much fun as a dental appointment. Good thing Harvey had come along to help push Nan's chair.

Harvey is Polish--that isn't his real name, just what he wants to be called. A motorcycle accident on the New Jersey Turnpike shortly after he arrived in the United States left him in a coma for eight years. The accident left him with a wide scar that parted his thinning blond hair, descended down his forehead and ended in his right eyebrow. Harvey was Chase's age but looked older. He lived three doors from Betsy and was her man-around-the-house, running errands, helping with chores, reading books and newspapers to her, and just being a human presence when she and Muffy felt lonely.

On the pavement next to Muffin sat an old army duffel bag filled with Nan's clean clothes: nightgowns, underwear, socks, handkerchiefs, towels, a robe, and a white satin bed jacket. Betsy had noticed things missing each time the Cedar Hills staff handled Nan's laundry, so she began taking it home with her. It would save time if she'd take the clothes inside to sort and put away while the others waited, but she was already tired and the day had just begun, Lord have mercy. She didn't want to add an extra trip inside to all the walking she'd have to do at Sea World.

*   *   *

At exactly eleven I parked the wheelchair van at the curb in front of Cedar Hills, fulfilling our on-time-or-early promise to customers. Betsy waved hello as I crossed the grass to the waiting group. "Oh boy," she said, when I got closer. "We must be pretty special to get the owner to drive for us."

I laughed. She said this every time I drove for her, tickled that I owned the company.

"Cathy's father died, his funeral is today. I hope you don't mind my filling in," I said after greeting her.

"How awful. Well of course we don't mind, dear. Glad to have you with us. You're going to tag along at Sea World I hope? Have lunch in the Harborside Restaurant? Our treat, naturally."

Before I could respond, a portly brown-skinned man in an ill-fitting safari suit said, "With a twenty-five dollar entrance fee each, Aunt Betsy, perhaps we should limit the number of people attending. Unless the driver wishes to pay her own way."

Before I could get an answer out, Betsy turned sharply and gave him a withering look, saying, "Butt out, Chase. Nanette is financing this little excursion." Muffin barked in agreement. Betsy bent at the waist to pick her up in one arm, soothing her with, "None of his business, is it Muffy?" The dog let loose a final yip.

To me she said, "We don't get rid of this five thousand dollars Nan inherited, she'll lose Medicare. You'd be doing us a favor if you'd come along, dear." Her mood lightened and she said, "Although I don't think we'll be able to spend it all today."

"I don't know, I have a pretty big appetite," I teased, and we both laughed.

She introduced me to Chase and Vashti. Harvey was always with Betsy, so I'd known him as long as I'd known her--four years. I shook Harvey's hand. He smiled and said, "Nice to see you again." And then, quietly, "If it's on sale I'll take a half pound of the sliced turkey." A byproduct of his long sleep was Harvey's often out-of-sync

211

responses. He might suddenly answer a question he'd been asked twenty minutes or two days earlier.

Once inside Betsy gestured to me and we fell behind the others, not difficult the way she slowly minced along; I only hoped I'd have half her strength in case I actually live to be ninety-two.

She took my arm and whispered, "Did you remember about the B12, dear? I'm pooped, and the day's just started, Lord have mercy. And my grand nephew is bugging me again to let his nerdy little wife take over my finances. Hurrumph."

I knew from prior conversations that Betsy handled all the financial matters for herself, Nan, and two other relatives also in rest homes. I can't balance my check book, so I was really impressed with this feat.

She squeezed my arm to communicate her urgency, and I almost cried out under her vise-like grip. I was half-a-foot taller, thirty pounds heavier--not to mention over fifty years younger--but I felt she could have wrestled me to the floor in an instant if she'd wanted to.

"Soon as that happened," she continued, "they'd move Nan to a cheaper rest home. One of those dumps where they bathe residents once a week, if that. Beatings. Neglect. Bed sores to the bone. Hurrumph." Her cane tapped smartly on the polished tile floor as she walked, keeping rhythm with the squeak of her Nikes. "Over my dead body."

*　　　*　　　*

The staff had dressed Nan in blue pajamas, blue silk robe and slippers; she was waiting in her wheelchair at the nurses station in section Rosewood. When Nan spotted us, she raised her arm and pointed a finger, saying, "Whirly, whirly, run whirly, *no*." Shouting now, "No no." She tried to get out of the chair, but the seatbelt kept her there. "Whiiiirly," she screamed in frustration, in a gravelly voice like a thousand fingernails across slate. "Run whirly."

Muffin raced down the hall toward Nan dragging her leash behind, nails clicking against the tiles. Nan's face softened and lost some of its terror as the dog approached. She ceased her struggle when Muffin sat down beside her footrest, tail buffing the already shiny floor. Nan reached down to stroke the dog's head.

212

"Yes whirly, run yes," she said in a quiet voice, and moved her hand to scratch behind Muffin's right ear.

Betsy was quick on Muffin's heels, moving down the brightly lit, gleaming hallway, in that tiny gait of hers--covering more ground than I would've believed possible with her mincing steps.

"Nan dear, its Bet," she called. "It's all right. I'm coming, Poodle. I'm coming."

Harvey stayed right beside Betsy the whole way. Chase was first at his grandmother's side, but didn't seem to know if he should embrace her. I hung back to give the family privacy. I was also not anxious to confront Nan in her present mood. On one outing to the San Diego Zoo, Betsy gave her a bunch of grapes to munch during the drive back to Cedar Hills. For every grape she ate, Nan pitched one at me, hitting my arm, shoulder, and the back of my head. It was all I could do not to pick them up and throw them back, I can be just as childish as the next person. Betsy scolded her, but didn't take the grapes. When I dropped them off, she apologized and gave me a fifty-dollar tip.

Vashti came to stand close to me; we looked at each other without speaking and her large brown eyes held a mixture of sadness and compassion. She was small, dark skinned, and reminded me of a younger, less-fiery version of Betsy.

We watched as Betsy cooed and fussed over Nan, smoothing her hair, patting her lined cheek. Nan's skin seemed to bear the age for both herself and Betsy, whose skin had sagged but was smooth as a rose petal. After a moment Nan looked directly at Betsy, seeming to recognize her, and smiling broadly, said, "Out going, run whirly?"

'Yes dear, that's right, we're going out. And we have company. Chase and Vashti are here." At this, Chase bent down and pecked her on the cheek. Nan reached up to lay her hand gently on the side of his face.

"And Harvey's here too." Betsy said, stepping back to reveal him. Nan stared as suspicion crossed her face.

"And Lynn's here to drive us to Sea World in one of her special vans. You know how you like that," Betsy said.

I knew from experience that Nan would either ignore me or raise her hackles immediately. Which was why Cathy was her regular driver; Nan even let Cathy feed her.

"Whirly, no no no no no!" she said, suddenly angry when I

stepped forward.

"Now Poodle, this is the Self Reliance girl," Betsy said, referring to the name of my company. You know you like Lynn," Betsy insisted.

"Where's Cathy?" Nan screamed, momentarily lucid, as she clawed the empty air in front of her with outstretched arms. Then, "Whirly, whirly no," she said before slumping back in her wheelchair.

Harvey took the initiative, pushing Nan's chair back the way we'd come. As we passed a water fountain I gestured to Betsy to stop while the others continued toward the exit. I gave her two 1000 microgram tablets of Vitamin B12, which she swallowed immediately with just a sip of water. At my urging she drank more.

"How long will it take to work?" Betsy asked. "Are you sure two are enough? They're such little things, maybe I should take more."

"In two hours I'll give you another two tablets, if you need them. You could start feeling better in less than an hour. Depends on your metabolism and digestive system."

"You're such a smart little thing," she said, and reached up to pat my cheek.

In the street, I lowered the lift to the asphalt and brought Nan's wheelchair down over the curb. I placed her on the lift, locking the brakes on both wheels and bracing my hip against the chair to keep it steady as we were lifted. After securing the wheelchair to the floor, I double checked Nan's seatbelt. Betsy sat next to me holding Muffin. Harvey took the jumpseat. Chase and Vashti followed in a rental car. Nan was quiet throughout, her eyes empty and unfocused.

*   *   *

Mission Bay is a tranquil green-blue inlet used for water recreation, less than fifteen minutes from downtown San Diego. It washes up on the community shores of Mission Beach to the west and Pacific Beach to the north, and is the site of the national Thunder Boat Races each September. Sea World sprawls across a hundred and fifty acre plot on one of the peninsulas floating in Mission Bay. Its three hundred foot sky tower, located in the center of the park, is an orientation point that can be seen for miles.

Strollers and wheelchairs are available to rent inside, to the right of the main entrance. Chase was already off to a bad start and didn't help himself when he volunteered to push Betsy if she wanted to rent a wheelchair. Too angry to answer, Betsy hobbled over and whacked him on the behind with her cane. I dropped down on one knee to fiddle with my shoestrings, trying to control the smile that was pasted to my face.

Chase was bewildered. "I was just trying to be helpful, Aunt Betsy," he said, rubbing his right cheek.

The blue sky was uninterrupted by clouds, the temperature a gentle seventy-two degrees. When we arrived at the park the sun was directly overhead, and a cool breeze was blowing off the bay. We were just in time for the sea lion and otter show, featuring Clyde and Seamore, who were marooned on an island. The outdoor show went for cheap wet laughs and the audience, mostly families with children, responded at all the right places. The two mammals seemed to genuinely enjoy themselves and eagerly gobbled up the fresh herring and mackerel offered after each feat.

During the show Betsy watched over Nan, several times wiping saliva from her chin. Each time Nan became briefly aware, reaching out lovingly to Betsy, saying, "Whirly whirly, run, run," or some like combination. Betsy told me Nan had been diagnosed with Alzheimer's ten years earlier, at 79, and her condition had deteriorated fast. She was now reduced to a vocabulary ordinarily consisting of five or six words and required full time care. Generally, her moods swung between rage and apathy, with small moments of lucidity sprinkled here and there as a kindness.

As we were leaving the stadium, filing out slowly with the crowd, I noticed a change in Betsy's mood. Her steps were perkier, and she raised her cane higher with each step, swinging it out before bringing it back to the asphalt. "Oh boy, wasn't that great?" she said to Harvey, who responded, "Yes, but I always pay my taxes on time."

A few minutes later we were seated on a bench near the dolphin pool, waiting for Chase and Vashti to return from the Catalina Grill with cold drinks, when Betsy asked me for more B12.

"This stuff is great, you betcha. I'm going to get a big bottle tomorrow morning first thing."

"You seem pretty energized to me already, Betsy. Looks like the B12 is working. Maybe you don't need anymore," I suggested.

"Nonsense. You said you had two more for me."

"If you *needed* them. If you don't, you shouldn't take anymore."

"I have a long day ahead of me *young* lady. And I don't intend to let Chase see me falter. Now fork 'em over. I like the way they make me feel."

I did as she asked, glancing at her cane. When the drinks arrived, she swallowed the tablets and winked at me. I just shook my head.

We fed the dolphins, and visited the shark encounter. On the way to see the penguins Chase complained that his feet hurt. He wanted to eat lunch before visiting any more attractions. I looked down; he was the only one not wearing athletic shoes. His tasseled loafers were designed for plush carpeting, not hot asphalt. He was adamant; he had missed lunch, he said. Betsy was just as determined to keep going, and decided to take a vote, counting Muffin and Nan on her side.

"Muffin is a dog. Grandmother is senile," Chase said with a sneer. "That means Vashti will have to break the tie."

"What about Lynn and Harvey?" Betsy asked.

"Lynn is hired help. And Harvey is almost as crazy as grandmother."

I was hoping Betsy would wallop him on the butt again, when Vashti's voice filled the stunned pause. "I agree with Chase," she said. "We should keep this in the family, and Chase's grandmother isn't competent to vote. I *should* break the tie."

We turned to face Vashti. Except for a quick hello when we first met, that was the first time I'd heard her voice. It was pleasant and melodic.

Nan screamed, "Whirly no!" at a passerby, who hastened away in the opposite direction.

Chase's sneer turned into a proud smile, which vanished with Vashti's next words. "I vote to keep walking and eat later, whenever Aunt Betsy thinks it's time."

Chase's mouth fell open. Betsy beamed at Vashti. My shoelaces needed attention again.

"Walk with me, Vashti. I've been meaning to talk to you about treasury, money-market trusts .... " Betsy said, as they sauntered off arm-in-arm.

We visited the forbidden reef, the bird showplace, and took in a Shamu & Friends killer whale show--watching the performance from a special glass-enclosed booth reserved for wheelchairs--before Betsy decided it was time to eat.

The Harborside Cafe is a full service, four star restaurant located on park grounds, with large windows overlooking Mission Bay. We were seated in time for the five o'clock water ski show, and we watched the performance while we ordered and waited for our food. All through dinner Chase complained--about the walking, about his aching joints, about his overdone steak, his under-baked potato. The sun had moved around and was directly on our table, another source of irritation for him. I thought the food was sensational. Harvey was so happy he was talking to his rice pilaf. Betsy fed Nan and said something nice each time Chase said something negative. He was way out of his league.

"Thank God we have to get grandmother back to Cedar Hills. Aunt Betsy would walk my butt into the ground otherwise. As it is, the exit is all the way on the other side of the park," Chase mumbled, as he spooned chocolate mousse into his mouth, smearing his moustache.

Vashti reached up with her napkin to wipe Chase's mouth at the same time Betsy reached up with hers to wipe Nan's. They caught sight of each other and laughed.

Betsy said to Chase. "Maybe we should ask them to bring a wheelchair over for you."

Chase actually considered it. Then laughter from Betsy and Vashti brought a scowl to his chubby face. I had a feeling life would never be the same for him.

CHAPTER 12

MAGNESIUM OXIDE

•Relieve Constipation Quickly, Safely, *Naturally*, And Forever
Ending Chronic Constipation
Ending Occasional Constipation *The Same Day*
Ending Occasional Constipation *Overnight*

Magnesium Oxide is a mineral, one of the vital compounds necessary for good health, which also include Calcium, Copper, Iodine, Iron, Manganese, Potassium, and Zinc, among others. Taken as directed, Magnesium Oxide can increase the amount of water retained in your food as it passes through your intestines during the digestive process, stopping constipation naturally. Constipation is simply a result of too much water being extracted during this process, leaving your feces dry, hardened, and difficult to pass.

Magnesium Oxide is a safe and effective alternative to treat occasional or chronic constipation. For example, during pregnancy many women experience constipation but are reluctant to use even over-the-counter drugs. Others who can benefit include elderly individuals who lead sedentary lives, those with paralysis, and people using antibiotics and other drugs that can cause constipation. Magnesium Oxide is fast acting and easy to digest, but *those with impaired kidney function should use it with caution, after consulting with their physician.*

Recommended Strength[28]

500 mg

Recommended Form

Tablets or capsules

Taken How

With eight ounces of juice or other liquids as directed.

Side Effects

None observed when taken as directed.

Notes√√

√ Since Magnesium Oxide causes your bowels to retain water, too much of the supplement can cause mild, short-term diarrhea that generally lasts for only one or two bowel movements.

√ Magnesium Oxide works interactively with other minerals, especially Calcium. If you are treating chronic constipation and taking Magnesium Oxide for more than a few days at a time, it is recommended that you also take a **Multiple Mineral** supplement. This will help prevent the depletion of other minerals that can lead to a different deficiency than the one being treated. If you are constipated infrequently and use Magnesium Oxide only occasionally, you do not have to take a Multiple Mineral. Whenever possible take the Multiple

---

28 The author has had the best results with <u>Schiff®</u> Magnesium Oxide, Salt Lake City, UT 84104, (800) 526-6251, available at most health foods stores and sometimes in the health foods section of supermarkets.

Mineral with Magnesium Oxide.

Multiple Mineral: Use in 500 mg chelated tablets or capsules.[29] The dosage strength is for Calcium only; the other Minerals will be present in varying amounts depending upon the formula. Take it with eight ounces of juice or other liquids as directed. If you do not use a chelated formula--one that is bound to amino acids--you may have to take it with food, because non-chelated formulas can be difficult to digest and assimilate.

1. Take 500 mg twice daily, morning and afternoon, and continue as a maintenance dose as long as you take Magnesium Oxide.

Remedy At A Glance (Multiple Mineral)

Daily As A Maintenance Dose While Taking Magnesium Oxide:	Morning	Afternoon
	500 mg	500 mg

See Volume II of this series for more on Multiple Minerals and how to use them to help prevent osteoporosis and trembling in your extremities.

•Relieve Constipation Quickly, Safely, *Naturally*, And Forever

Ending Chronic Constipation

1. Take 500 mg of Magnesium Oxide, three times daily, morning, afternoon, and evening, and continue for one week.

2. Reduce to 500 mg twice daily, morning and afternoon, and

---

29 The author has had the best results with Nature's Life® Vegetarian Mega Minerals, Garden Grove, CA 92841, (800) 854-6837, available at most health foods stores and sometimes in the health foods section of supermarkets.

continue for four weeks.

3. Reduce to 500 mg once a day in the morning, and continue as a maintenance dose to help prevent constipation.

Remedy At A Glance (Magnesium Oxide)

	Morning	Afternoon	Evening
Daily For One Week To Relieve Constipation:	500 mg	500 mg	500 mg
Daily For Four Weeks To Relieve Constipation:	500 mg	500 mg	
Daily As A Maintenance Dose:	500 mg		

Notes √√

√ If you experience diarrhea at any time while you are taking Magnesium Oxide, reduce your daily intake by eliminating one dosage. If necessary, continue to *decrease* the daily dosage until you reach your own comfort level.

√ If this protocol does not fully relieve your constipation, double one or more of the doses to 1000 mg, or increase the frequency of the 500 mg doses. If necessary, continue to *increase* the daily dosage slowly--in small increments over a number of days--until you reach your own comfort level.

√ If you are not in any of the groups mentioned at the top of the chapter--pregnant, sedentary elderly, paralysis disabled, or taking antibiotics or other drugs that can cause constipation--your problem may be diet related. Some foods that can be very effective in helping to relieve and prevent constipation are: any kind of cooked dried pea or bean,[30] fresh papaya, mango, pear, and apple, mixed salad vegetables,

---

[30] Leave the top off the pot or prop it open while the peas or beans are cooking. The indigestible sugars will cook off in the steam, eliminating the gaseous episodes associated with eating these foods.

and freshly-squeezed carrot juice. Consumed daily, these foods can help keep you regular.

√ Another food source very effective in preventing constipation is edible **Aloe Vera Gel.**[31]

Aloe Vera Gel: Use in liquid form. Take it on an empty stomach in the middle of the day, followed by eight ounces of water. It has a blandly pleasant taste, but can be mixed with water or other liquids if you prefer.

1. Take one tablespoon once a day, and continue as a maintenance dose to help prevent constipation.

Remedy At A Glance (Aloe Vera Gel)

	On An Empty Stomach Followed By 8 oz Water
Daily As A Maintenance Dose:	One Tablespoon

√ If your constipation is accompanied by gas in your stomach or intestines, it is recommended that you also take **Activated Charcoal,** which can relieve gas throughout the digestive tract.

Activated Charcoal: Use 260 mg strength (4 grain), capsules only.[32] Take it with juice or other liquids as directed.

1. Take 520 mg after each meal, if you suffer from chronic gas discomfort.

2. Take 520 mg at first sign of discomfort, if you have gas only occasionally.

31-32 For both edible Aloe Vera Gel liquid, and Activated Charcoal, the author has had the best results with <u>Puritan's Pride®</u>, Oakdale, NY 11769, available by mail order only at (800) 645-1030.

3. You may take 520 mg every two hours as needed to relieve occasional gas, up to four doses in one day. If this daily amount is not enough to relieve your gas discomfort, you should contact a physician to ensure that nothing is seriously wrong with your digestive tract.

Remedy At A Glance (Activated Charcoal)

Daily To Relieve Symptoms:	After Each Meal For Chronic Gas Discomfort	As Needed For Occasional Gas Discomfort
	520 mg	520 mg

Ending Occasional Constipation
The Same Day

1. Take 1000 mg of Magnesium Oxide in the morning, and 1000 mg in the afternoon.

2. If necessary, take 500 mg in the early evening.

3. If your constipation occurs in the latter part of the day, follow the instructions below for relieving it overnight.

Remedy At A Glance (Magnesium Oxide)

To Relieve Constipation Same Day:	Morning	Afternoon	Early Evening If Necessary
	1000 mg	1000 mg	500 mg

Ending Occasional Constipation *Overnight*

1. Take 1000 mg of Magnesium Oxide in the afternoon, and 1000 mg in the evening.

Remedy At A Glance (Magnesium Oxide)

To Relieve	Afternoon	Evening
Constipation Overnight:	1000 mg	1000 mg

Notes√√

√ Expect to make a trip to the bathroom as soon as you wake up. If the urge disturbs your sleep prematurely during the night, take the evening dose later, i.e., an hour before bedtime.

*   *   *

The following is a case study written as a short story about one of countless people who have been helped by this remedy: A pregnant magazine editor in New York City faces an important deadline and finds grateful relief with Magnesium Oxide when over-the-counter medications fail.

"The Crocodile And The Goose"

Maria Rosa Isabella Corras Gonzalez's voice was a small plea, as she stalked the aisles between the four-foot-high partitioned cubicles housing the staff of Steiner-Hampton Publishing on Manhattan's lower east side.

"Let's go, people," she said under her breath. "Less than eight hours to pick-up."

She was a junior editor, and the first five issues of her magazine had not done as well as expected; advertisers were dropping out. The sixth, and last-if-the-numbers-didn't-improve, issue was due at the Missouri printer tomorrow afternoon.

And there were problems.

The paste-up artists were still making corrections to galleys and mechanicals, and cleaning adhesive from boards; photostats were being reshot to comply with lay-outs the art director kept changing; captions were two picas wider than the specs and were being reset. Color was off on the advance copy of the cover: The bride's white satin brocade gown was the same blue as the thinning hair of her elderly aunts back in Rio Piedras. Yellow bridesmaid's dresses were the color of guacamole, and their complexions suggested they needed oxygen immediately. And she was still waiting on line art from two freelance illustrators.

Perhaps worst of all, Maria had been constipated for weeks, hadn't gone at all in three days. Bloated, cramped with painful gas, she was six feet of misery, midway through her seventh month with her first baby weighing heavily on her lower body. For some reason her physician couldn't explain, over-the-counter remedies didn't work. She was afraid to take anything stronger for fear it could harm the baby.

Maria had started as a typesetter in the magazine division in 1978, a month after moving to New York from Puerto Rico. She left her husband of three years on the island, not because there were problems with the marriage, but because she was professionally stifled. Women were still confined to "traditional" jobs, and advancement into management, or advancement of any kind, almost always went to men. Maria was passed over repeatedly, and when another man she trained was promoted over her, she quit. Before going home that day, she drove to San Juan International Airport and bought a ticket to the mainland. She loved Puerto Rico, it was her motherland. But she was certain if she stayed she would never live out her dreams. After two years setting type, she was promoted to copyediting. Another year passed before Sally Hampton gave her *Brides & Bridesmaids* to edit, a real coup her first time out, eighty pages with sixteen in color, the most of any but the automotive titles.

Maria continued winding through the cubicles, working her way toward reception and the administrative offices, greeting other staffers as she passed. In the automotive section an editor was mouthing off to a contributor twice his size; dressed in black leather, she looked angry enough to hurt the editor bad; she also looked plenty capable. In the interior design grouping they were comparing fabric swatches of chintz and linen for a drapery lay out in an art-deco spread. Health and beauty, nearest the front offices, had six people jammed into a cubicle to assist in a facial. The overheard conversations were like small tributaries emptying into a river of sound; Maria reveled in the constant flow of activity in the big room.

She picked up the deliveries in the front and turned to start back to her office, noting the reflection that bounced back from the glass

226

doors leading out of reception. Oval face, oak-brown skin, black eyes, freckles on her nose and cheeks, black shoulder length hair. She was wearing a denim granny dress, long sleeved with an empire waist and lots of room in the skirt. Because her ankles were swollen like summer apples, she wore only white Tretorn sneakers with assorted colors of slouch socks.

Around the periphery on three sides were private and semi-private offices, mostly occupied by management, senior editors, and the art director's suite. Junior editors, graphic artists, typesetters, copy editors, researchers, and proofreaders occupied the partitioned cubicles in the enormous center of the windowless room. The outside world could be glimpsed through windows in offices visible through open doorways. The view today showed a morning that awoke under a shroud of gray haze and washed its face with September showers, while the rumble of thunder across the tops of skyscrapers made occupants flinch.

The baby kicked at that moment, reminding her she had forgotten to ask Michael to order breakfast. The very next instant she was famished. Her hunger escalated as she closed in on her office, until she thought she could actually smell the breakfast sandwich she ordered each morning. It wasn't on the restaurant's menu, but since getting pregnant she had been ordering four or five times a day, so they indulged her. It wasn't her imagination, for sitting in the middle of her desk was a sandwich made with three strips of crisp bacon, two sunny-sides, and a slice of American cheese on buttered rye toast spread with strawberry jam. Hash browns were on the side. Pink grapefruit juice waited patiently in tall Styrofoam.

"Ohhh, Michael, *gracias a Dios*," she groaned, as she fell on the food, tearing open the wrappers and filling her mouth with large bites like a starving wolf. The eggs were heavily peppered and made the yolks tantalizingly hot. She moaned out loud when the taste exploded against her tongue. She felt as though she hadn't eaten in days, instead of the two hours that had passed since she'd had a decaf mocha latte, two chocolate doughnuts, a butter croissant, and two bagels generously frosted with creme cheese. Michael was talking to her, but Maria was too hungry to listen, could hear only the sounds of her own chewing and her stomach sighing in anticipation. When he walked away shaking his head, she said with her mouth full, "Sorry, Michael. *Momemtito.*" She held up her right hand, with thumb and index half-an-inch apart, to indicate she would be with him shortly.

Michael left Maria to enjoy her food and crossed to a darkened corner of her office. It was kept that way, with blinds closed, to create the proper environment for the waist-high light box--fluorescent tubes set inside a metal box four feet by two, with an opaque sheet of glass covering the top. He clicked the switch and watched the lights flicker and dance to life, then placed three rows of color transparencies on the glass. Maria would choose one of them for next month's cover--if there was one. It had to be mocked up for color and copy and sent to the printer in one week, regardless. They could always pull it off the schedule later. He bent over the light box to examine each transparency through a loop, a small eight-power magnifier shaped like an upside-down shot glass.

While Maria chewed the last of the potatoes and sucked the final drops of juice through a straw, she looked out the large windows of her office, grateful to be of one of the few junior editors with her own space. She could see into the windows of the building across from her, where other people worked diligently on tasks and dealt with crises that meant nothing to her and everything to them. She knew people looking back felt the same. Each floor of lights was a bright planet of activity snuggled away from the damp gray atmosphere. She finished her food and sat back in the cushy swivel chair, fighting the urge to take a nap. It was 9:00 a.m.

Michael closed the door and sat down across the desk from her, crossing his legs with one ankle on top of the other knee. As usual, his expression was neutral. His squared face could have been contemplating nuclear devastation or deciding which vegetable to choose for dinner. He was 28, tall and lanky, a second generation Chinese-American whose grandparents had immigrated to the United States from Nanyuan. He wore a beige dress shirt with sleeves rolled to the elbow, no tie, black vest, Levi's, and Reeboks. Straight black hair covered his ears and hung past his neck.

Maria sat straighter, trying to revive her sluggish mind, and heard an obscene growling noise crash against the leather as she accidentally passed gas.

"Excuse me," she said in a small, embarrassed voice.

Michael pretended to be too interested in his notes to notice, even when the sulfurous aroma passed under his nose. Maria's intestines felt as though she were carrying bricks in them. She was so uncomfortable she wanted to scream, but she gave Michael her full attention when he began speaking.

"First, Elaine called in sick, has the flu, can't put the book to bed this afternoon."

Maria's eyes widened, and she gripped the arms of the chair.

"I've already arranged for a freelance art director to take over for the next couple of days. Okay? So calm down. Called Jim Braid over at Hearst to see if Lynn was available. Luckily, they're between projects for the next two weeks. She'll be here by ten. You've met her before, last year I think, she spent a couple of weeks working with the automotive department on their titles. Cliff said she's real good."

"Michael, I swear, if I weren't already married you would not be safe from me. Promise you will never leave me," Maria joked. She spoke in a slow, velvety contralto, almost a monotone, with only some words accented with the rhythm of her native Spanish.

"You're welcome. And I promise to never leave you."

Michael had taken the job as Maria's secretary/assistant, even though it meant a twenty percent pay cut, because he was interested in editing children's books. She promised to help him get his own title after he'd learned the ropes. It didn't take him long to discover he was falling in love with her. Within a month of meeting Maria, he was moping through weekends in anticipation of the start of a new work week.

Reinvigorated by the ease with which the near catastrophe had been averted, Maria rubbed her palms together and asked, "What's next?"

Michael glanced at the framed picture of Maria's husband, Tony, sitting on a shelf behind her. A close up showing a broad face and fullback shoulders, cinnamon-color skin, white teeth, jeweled earring in left lobe, wearing a grey cashmere v-neck. Cocky conceit written all over his face. He had finally moved to New York to be with Maria but still spent several months a year in San Juan running a boat repair business. Michael couldn't be sure whether he disliked Tony because of who he was, or because of his own feelings for Maria. He suspected a little of both. Likewise, he wished he could be sure that he was telling her now because it was the right thing to do, not because he dreamed of getting Tony out of her life.

"How long have you and Tony been married again?" he asked, trying his best to sound casual, hoping the anxiety in his heart wasn't betrayed by his voice.

Maria relied on Michael to keep her steady. His equanimity was her port in any storm. Now that his usually placid features sketched apprehension, she felt her heart skip to a faster pace. He always laid things out in such a forthright manner, that now her blood chilled with the wonder of what he had to say that was so bad he had to build up to it. *Madre de Dios.*

"Seven years in December. I was twenty-three," said Maria.

They stared at each other for a long time without speaking.

"Miiiiichael," she said, dragging out his name. "You're scaring me. Did someone call from the island? Did something happen to Tony?"

"No. Nothing like that. Don't upset yourself."

"Then what is it? Forgodsake."

Michael shifted in his seat and took a deep breath, saying, "My grandmother tells a story to the young children in my family, told to her by her grandmother, and so forth," he began, speaking slowly. "About a crocodile and a goose who had a good friendship. One lovely spring day, under a low hanging tree, they languished lazily in the warm waters of a slow-moving river."

Maria rolled her eyes. "Can't you just tell me what you know?"

Michael stared at her hard, before he cleared his throat and continued in an even voice. "The crocodile stayed in the thick mud near the shore, while the goose swam in circles just at the edge of the shade. The crocodile kept the goose's company, because she was good with a turn of phrase, and he had spent many pleasurable afternoons listening to her recount one of her fables.

" 'Well, my fine fat goose,' cried the crocodile. 'What amusement do you have for my consideration today?'

"The goose was very flattered by the crocodile's attention, and each time they met she did indeed endeavor to capture his interest with one of the engaging stories she'd heard during her travels up shore. She was sure he would be equally charmed by today's tale:

"The goose ruffled her white feathers dramatically and began, 'Once upon a time, deep within a lush green forest, there was an ivy-covered glen where there dwelled the people of Orange ....'

For the next half hour she spun a tale of such delight and

cheerful enchantment that the crocodile remained utterly enthralled, listening closely, and slapping his tail merrily when it particularly pleased him, splattering mud on the goose's fine feathers in the process, though she thought it best not to complain."

Michael's voice deepened as he warmed to his tale, and took on a story teller's quality, rising for the hills and dropping into the valleys. He felt himself relax and was certain he was doing the right thing in the right way.

"While he liked the telling of the tale, the crocodile was unhappy with the ending. 'I don't blame the hero for being a bit disgusted,' the crocodile said matter-of-factly, and stretched his short legs in the muddy water.

" 'Ohhh, I'm afraid you have quite entirely missed the moral of the story,' scolded the goose.

" 'What!' flared the crocodile. 'You dared tell me a story with a moral? I certainly didn't come here to be preached to by the likes of you.'

"And before he knew what he was doing, the crocodile had gobbled the goose whole, and she did make a rare and tasty repast, right down to her last Honk! of surprise. The crocodile was immediately saddened by the loss of his dear friend, for he would miss her fine storytelling. But really, she ought to have known better."

Michael finished and waited.

The silence stretched and was shattered by the ringing telephone. Michael jumped, but Maria sat as if in a trance, staring down at her desk top.

"The art director is here," Michael said, after answering it. "She's early, want me to get her started while you think about what I just said?"

"I have no idea what the hell you just said."

"Well, maybe you do and maybe you don't. We can talk about it after I get Lynn set up in Elaine's office. I'll be right back. Don't move."

No problem. Maria was glued to her seat. She didn't understand what Michael was trying to tell her, but she couldn't completely convince herself of this, because something tickled her mind, as if she had just awakened from a dream with all the emotion but none of the memory.

231

Michael returned after twenty minutes. "Lynn says she doesn't see any problem bringing it all together by four," he said, as he came through the door.

Anxious to get to the bottom of Michael's parable, Maria said, "First explain the moral of the crocodile eating the goose. I don't get it. Why did he do it? Weren't they good friends? Didn't he miss her as soon as he gobbled her up? What was the point? Her friendship had to mean more than that moment of pleasure he got from eating her. Was he even hungry?"

"The point is, that even though the goose could trust the crocodile, because they were good friends, in the end she could only trust him to be a crocodile," Michael said, praying she would understand without more information from him.

Maria's bladder was full, and she could barely sit straight because of the tremendous pressure of gas in her intestines. "I have to go to the bathroom. When I get back I want it straight out. You hear me? No more fairy tales."

When she returned with her bladder emptied but still feeling completely unrelieved, a spot on her desk had been cleared; in the center of the space was an envelope. When Maria sat down she saw it was a phone bill from a mobile service.

"What's this?" she asked, without making a move to touch it.

"It's the bill from Tony's new cell phone carrier. It was sent here by mistake."

Maria stared at the envelope for a long time. Michael waited, unwilling to volunteer any more right now.

"Tony's the crocodile, right?" she finally asked in a quiet voice. "Guess that makes me the *fine fat goose*. Perfect analogy. Thanks a lot."

"I'm sorry. I didn't mean it that way. I think you're beautiful with life stirring inside you." He said it too fast, and his voice carried more emotion than he intended to reveal.

Maria wasn't prepared to deal with what she heard in Michael's voice or saw in his eyes at that moment. She said, "Come on, tell me the rest. What did my nasty crocodile do?"

Michael decided to give it all to her. "I was on my way to the Registrar's office to sign up for fall classes a couple of weeks ago. I saw Tony on campus. I didn't think anything about it until I came to work the next day and you told me how much you missed him because he was in San Juan that week. Then the next day, I'm on campus again to get a professor to sign my registration card. I stopped at a coffee shop on West Fourth when I was through. He was there--with another woman." He cleared his voice before continuing, watching Maria closely for any reaction. "You could see from their behavior that they were ... that they had been ... *together*."

Again Michael waited.

Maria sat still as stone, eyes on the envelope.

"What's this have to do with it," she asked, indicating the phone bill with a thrust of her chin.

"I opened it thinking it was your bill. Discovered Tony'd established a separate account in his own name. Because I was worried about what I'd seen on campus, I did a little investigating, especially after I noticed that most of the outgoing calls were going to three numbers."

"Where'd they ring at?" Maria finally looked up at Michael who was standing in front of her desk with both hands shoved in the rear pockets of his black jeans.

One rings at French House on NYU's campus, another goes to Bobst Library. One is for a private residence. I got an answering machine. A woman's voice."

"Which number got the answering machine?" Maria asked, picking up the receiver.

She punched in the numbers Michael gave her and listened to a young female voice ask her to leave the time, date, and a short message. There was a pause followed by static, then, "Tony, class is canceled tonight. I'll see you at Harold's at eight."

Maria replaced the receiver and leaned her head back against the worn leather, too stunned to cry, feeling a large empty hole opening up inside her.

*   *   *

I pushed in the door to the ladies room and was struck by the unsettling sound of someone crying. Seated on a green Naugahyde divan in the outer chamber was a pregnant woman, making no pretense at hiding her misery. I passed her without comment and went into the next room where the stalls were located, wanting to respect her privacy.

233

While washing my hands, I realized it was Maria Gonzalez, my editor. She had a private office, so why was she venting in public? I stopped to console her on my way out, just a tiny bit curious about what could be important enough to distract her from today's deadline.

I touched her shoulder, saying, "Maria, are you okay? Can I get you anyth ... "

She turned around suddenly, wrapping her arms around my legs, leaning into me for comfort, and really cutting loose with the sobs. I held her and rubbed her back. After a while I said, "Let me take you back to your office, Maria, we can talk for a few minutes. Until you calm down. The magazine is under control, really, if that's what's worrying you."

She pulled away from me, shaking her head. "I can't ... can't let Michael see me like this. He'll feel bad for telling me, but I'm glad he told me. I would rather know the tr .... " She began to stutter and her words were swallowed by another outpouring of tears.

"But ... if someone sees you in here like this, won't it get back to Michael anyway?"

This made sense, and she nodded, taking a deep breath before going into the next room to wash her face.

Michael was nowhere to be seen, so we closed her office door and sat on a couch facing a window. Like most people who find out a spouse or partner is cheating, a lot of things too small to notice before the discovery made perfect sense after it: She remembered the phone calls with no one at the other end--when she answered. How Tony had stopped eating dinner at home a couple of nights a week, saying he wasn't hungry because of a large lunch, when he'd packed only sandwiches that day. The times he had come home from work, showered and dressed sharp, even putting on cologne--just to hang out with the guys. And Sunday afternoons, a time they always saved for each other. Gone, because Tony had joined a gym on the other side of town and spent the whole afternoon "working out", instead of cuddling in bed, eating cinnamon rolls, and reading the *Sunday Times* together. She said at the end, "He was working out alright."

When she finished her account of Tony the louse, she said, "And I'm going to explode if I can't go to the bathroom. I am sooo uncomfortable. Been constipated for weeks."

"I can't help you with your marital problems, but I can help you with that," I said, and went to her desk for pen and paper.

"There's a health-foods store on Third Avenue on the corner of 23rd Street, just a few blocks from here. Can you get someone to go? You want to buy Magnesium Oxide. Here," I indicated the paper. "I've written it all down. It's a mineral, only takes a couple of hours to start working. Oh yeah. If you have gas, ask the person to buy Activated Charcoal as well."

*   *   *

I gave the package to the Fed Ex agent at exactly four o'clock, for the overnight shipment to the printer. I straightened my area, cleared off the drafting table, cleaned the art tools and put them back where they belonged. I had brought my own compass and template set, X-acto knife, and flexible curve, which I returned to my large portfolio case.

Maria had sent a messenger for the supplements and taken them right away. I got busy after that and didn't see her again for several hours. Curious now to find out if the Magnesium Oxide had relieved her discomfort, I went to her office. I found Michael there, repeating the actions I'd just performed, straightening her desk and work area. He told me she hadn't been out of the bathroom in the last hour.

Just then she came waddling in, cheeks flushed, with a look of ecstasy on her face usually seen only on the features of enraptured religious statuary.

"I take it the Magnesium Oxide worked?"

"Boy, did it ever," she said." "How can I ever thank you?"

"Don't worry about it. I'm glad you feel better. The look on your face is payment enough," I said, laughing.

She laughed and joked with me until the urge struck her again in a few minutes.

"Oops, gotta' go," she said, and headed back to the bathrooms.

CROSS REFERENCE OF CONDITIONS TREATED IN VOLUME I

Conditions and Chapters[33]

A

Age Spots, **3**
Allergies, **7**, 5, 9
Alzheimers, **2**
Aneurism Stroke, **10**
Angina Pain, **9**, 5
Arteriosclerosis, **9**, 5
Arthritis, **9**, 3, 5, 7, 11
Asthma, **3**, 5, 9

B

Bleeding Gums, **10**
Bloodclot Stroke, **9**, 5
Bloodshot Eyes, **10**
Blocked Arteries, **9**, 5
Breathing Problems, **3**
Breast Fibroids, **5**

Bronchitis, **3**, 5, 9
Bruising, **10**
Bursitis, **5**
Blocked Heart Valve, **9**, 5

C

Cancer Generally, **5**
Cigarette Smoker's Damage, **3**
Cold Sores, **4**
Colds, **7**, 5, 9
Colon Cancer, **5**, 8
Congestion, **9**
Constipation, **12**
Crohn's Disease, **5**, 8

D

Decreased Circulation, **11**

Diarrhea Generally, **8**
Discolored Toenails, **8**

E

Exposure to Pollution, **3**
Exposure to Second-Hand Smoke, **3**
Exposure to Toxins, **3**

F

Fatigue, **6**, 11
Fatty Deposits In Liver, **9**
Feminine Itching, **8**
Flu, **4**, 5, 9, 11

---

[33] For page numbers where each disorder is discussed, please consult the Index. Bolded numbers indicate chapters where the remedy for that condition is featured. Other numbers indicate chapters for additional supplements, which are recommended to enhance the primary remedy. For more information on any chapter, please consult the Table of Contents on page ix.

INDEX

240

Mental Exhaustion, 7-9, 11-12
Mental Fatigue, 7-9, 11-12
Mineral Deposits, 149-152,
    157-158
Minerals, 111, 219-221
Minor Injury, 69-71, 79-80
Morning Fatigue, 197-199,
    201-202
Multiple Minerals, 220-221

N

Nagging Cough, 21-24, 25-28,
    69-71, 74, 76-78, 149-152,
    156-157
Nature's Food Farm Brand, 151
Nature's Life Brand, 221
Niacin (B3), 197
Nosebleeds, 179-181, 184
NOW Brand, 8

O

Osteoarthritis, 149-152, 158-159

P

Panic Attack, 91-94
Panic Disorders, 91-94
Pantothenic Acid (B5), 197
Para-Aminobenzoic Acid
    (PABA), 197
Performance Anxiety, 91-94
Phosphatides, 151
Piper Methysticum, 54, 93
Pollution Exposure, 21-24, 37
Potassium, 219
Preparation For And Recovery
    From Surgery, 69-71, 73
Promoting A Healthy
    Cardiovascular System, 69-71,
    74, 149-156, 179-183
Promoting A Healthy Intestinal
    Tract, 133-135, 139-141,
219-225
Promoting Healthy Blood Vessels,
    179-185
Promoting Healthy Gums,
    179-181, 184-185
Promoting Healthy Joints, 69-71,
    74, 149-152, 158-165,
Promoting Healthy Lungs, 21-32
Promoting Leg Vein Health,
    179-184
Protection From Pollution, 21-24,
    37
Protection From Environmental
    Toxins, 21-24, 37
Protein Deposits, 149-152,
    157-158
Puritan's Pride Brand, 8, 10, 23,
    52, 70, 75, 96, 112, 115, 134,
    151, 156, 180, 199
Pyridoxine (B6), 197

R

Reaction To Antibiotics, 133-135,
    140-141, 219-225,
Reduced Scarring, 69-73, 79-80
Repetitive Stress Disorder, 69-71,
    74
Respiratory Illnesses, 21-32,
    69-71, 74, 76-78
Rheumatoid Arthritis, 69-71, 74,
    149-152, 160-165
Riboflavin (B2), 197,
Ruptured Facial Capillaries,
    179-181, 184
Rutin, 22, 32, 111, 179-182, 184

S

Saturated Fats,
    protection when eating
    them, 149-152, 157-158